MEDICINE, ETHICS AND THE LAW

AUSTRALIA AND NEW ZEALAND
The Law Book Company
Sydney : Melbourne : Perth

CANADA AND U.S.A.
The Carswell Company Ltd.
Agincourt, Ontario

INDIA
N. M. Tripathi Private Ltd.
Bombay
and
Eastern Law House Private Ltd.
Calcutta and Delhi
M.P.P. House
Bangalore

ISRAEL
Steimatzky's Agency Ltd.
Jerusalem : Tel Aviv : Haifa

MEDICINE, ETHICS AND THE LAW

CURRENT LEGAL PROBLEMS

Edited by

M. D. A. Freeman, LL.M.

Professor of English Law at the University of London

London
Stevens & Sons
1988

Published in 1988
by Stevens & Sons Ltd.
of 11 New Fetter Lane, London
Laserset by P.B. Computer Typesetting, Pickering, N. Yorks.
Printed in Great Britain

British Library Cataloguing in Publication Data

Freeman, M.D.A. (Michael David Alan), 1943–
Medicine, ethics and the law. — (Current
legal problems).
1. England.   Medicine.   Law
I. Title   II. Series
344.204'41

ISBN 0–420–48020–X

PREFACE

This is the sixth special issue of *Current Legal Problems* to appear. It is the first to be based on a series of seminars. These were held in October and November 1987. All seven contributors read prepared papers, after which valuable debate ensued. The papers are reproduced here, more or less in the form that they were given.

University College is particularly grateful to those who gave papers and to other distinguished participants who gave of their time. In particular, I would like to thank Dr. Raanan Gillon, the editor of the *Journal of Medical Ethics*, Dr. John Havard and Dr. John Dawson of the British Medical Association, Chris Heginbotham, the Director of MIND and Professor Christina Lyon of Keele University who were kind enough to agree to chair sessions, as well as a number of colleagues who helped me run the seminars, particularly whilst I laboured with the handicap of a broken leg. Bob Hepple, Ian Dennis, Dawn Oliver, Rodney Austin and Isobel Gurney deserve especial mention. The preparation of a series like this involved a lot of work which was rendered the easier with Suzy Hoey's able assistance. To her also I am extremely grateful.

M.D.A. Freeman
January 1, 1988

CURRENT LEGAL PROBLEMS SPECIAL ISSUES

CONTENTS

TABLE OF CASES

Table of Cases

TABLE OF STATUTES

Introduction: Legal and Philosophical Frameworks for Medical Decision-Making

M.D.A. FREEMAN

This special issue of *Current Legal Problems* is the first to emerge from a series of staff seminars. The seminars, seven in all, took place in the Autumn term of 1987.

The interface between law, medicine and philosophy which, in different ways, each of the essays in this volume explores is indubitably one of the most significant of current legal problems.[1] Science, in particular but not exclusively bio-technology, has given doctors tools to work miracles, to cause life and to prolong it. The ethical dilemmas to which this gives rise are both manifold and intractable.[2] Decision-making cannot be governed by consensus for clearly there is none. There may be agreement on such fundamental principles as the sanctity of life but conflict remains on the content to be attached to such a principle. Many who oppose abortion favour capital punishment.[3] The ultimate decisions cannot be left to doctors alone. But doctors are expected to provide answers. Lawyers and philosophers can debate the questions involved endlessly, but doctors must take decisions, often there and then.

They work within the framework of the law. In Britain this is largely the common law because Parliament has not found it easy to legislate in these sensitive areas. The Abortion Act of 1967 and the Surrogacy Arrangements Act of 1985, the former now a largely-discredited compromise which has failed to provide answers to problems raised by new techniques,[4] the latter a largely irrelevant panicked measure,[5] are the two main examples of statutory intervention. The Human Tissue Act 1961 is a third example. But there have been many more attempts to legislate which have foundered because of profound moral conflict.[6] There are areas in which legislation is urgently needed (for example, to regulate embryo research, a fact recognised by the Government in

1

a White Paper[7] published after the conclusion of the seminars):
there are others in which control through self-regulation may be
preferable, codes published by the British Medical Association or
guidance by the Voluntary Licensing Authority. But these too can
give rise to controversy, as witness the *Gillick*[8] saga or the conflict
in 1987 between the VLA and the Humana Wellington Hospital
on the number of pre-embryos transferred to the woman's uterus
and on ovum donation between sisters and other close relatives.[9]
A statutory licensing authority, as advocated in the recent White
Paper,[10] may have more clout, but is unlikely to eliminate such
conflict. Even where there is legislation it is surprising to discover
how many issues of moral controversy remain. Thus, despite, or
arguably because of,[11] legislation on mental health,[12] the question
as to whether anyone could give consent to a mentally handicapped adult being sterilised fuelled the fires of controversy in 1987[13]
and still remains a matter of profound legal and moral concern. It
is reflected in two of the papers in this volume.[14]

But working within the framework of the common law is itself
fraught with problems. Many of the issues thrown up by biomedical advances elude the ingenuity or the skills of lawyers.
Precedent has an important role to play in areas of property and
commerce, but often seems to obstruct solutions where novel
ethical questions are posed. It is by nature a conservative doctrine
and the reference back of new problems to old concepts, practices
and institutions often can have a distorting effect. We can stretch
the law of adoption (the ban on money changing hands, for
example) to encompass surrogacy arrangements[15] or the law of
perpetuities to embrace the stored frozen embryo (*en ventre sa
mère* seemingly becoming *en ventre sa frigidaire!*)[16] but are we wise
to do so? Lord Reid did not have matters as contentious as these in
mind when, in 1969, he distinguished "lawyer's law" from "cases
which directly affect the lives and interests of large sections of the
community and on which laymen are as well able to decide as are
lawyers"[17] but in his terms the problems spawned by medical
developments would come into the latter category and show, in
effect, how facile the distinction is, for who could pretend that lay
persons are as well able to find solutions to the questions on the
margins of life and death that now confront us? The limits of the
common law are well-illustrated in Andrew Grubb's essay: but the
limits of alternatives are also all too painfully obvious. If the courts
have reached an impasse on such matters as informed consent or
on what should be compensated when a sterilisation operation
fails, who is to step into the breach? Are these matters we can
entrust to a legislature without the assistance of a research and

reform body? And is the Law Commission, the usual remit of such
tasks, composed as it is solely of lawyers, an appropriate forum for
the debates involved? It has itself, on previous occasions, admitted
that it can offer us more than a "field of choice,"[18] and we may
doubt whether on the profound moral questions raised by medical
progress it would necessarily even choose the correct field.

It is difficult to see a legal route out of this "moral quagmire."
The establishment of a standing commission, composed of
lawyers, doctors, philosophers, theologians and other disciplines,
as advocated by Ian Kennedy[19] is part, perhaps an important part,
of the answer. But the creation of structures is only as valuable as
the expertise contained within them. Of course, inter-professional
collaboration is important. "No man is an island," and we can all
profit from the insights of other disciplines, as those of us who
attended the seminars constantly found. Genuine inter-
professional debate is not easy to attain, a fact testified to by
anyone who has read the reports of inquiries into child deaths from
Colwell[20] to Carlile[21] and Henry.[22] There is always the danger that
it can lead to a broadening, but not a sharpening, of responsibility.

It is as well to be reminded that the problems confronting us in
Britain are shared by the medical and legal professions as well as
the philosophers of other countries.[23] The transplantation of
solutions to ethical problems is far from straightforward but,
where the countries have approximately similar cultures and
philosophies, we should not ignore the work done in them. The
Dutch experience with euthanasia legislation,[24] New Zealand's
with no fault liability (discussed in Sheila McLean's paper, based
on her own research in New Zealand),[25] the USA's with a
compulsory sterilisation programme, which I discuss, are all
valuable pointers. The Canadian Supreme Court decision in *Re
Eve*,[26] the "Baby M" surrogacy litigation,[27] the US and Common-
wealth case law on wrongful life (analysed in Grubb's essay) the
Quinlan[28] and *Bouvia*[29] cases are precedents we should study, if
only to profit from the mistakes of others.

The law is an indispensable framework but it is not some neutral
tool wielded in an apolitical way by disinterested players. It is very
much a social product, a reflection of the power of particular
interest groups, economic, religious and professional. The political
economy of decision-making in the area of medical law comes
sharply into focus when health resource allocation is questioned,[30]
as happened in two widely-published affairs during the period of
the seminars. In the *Harriott* case,[31] an ex-prostitute, denied IVF
treatment because of her history, unsuccessfully sought judicial
review of the decision to take her off the programme. In the affair

over a "hole-in-the-heart" operation for a six-week-old baby,[32] litigation was brought (once again unsuccessfully) to force the hands of the health authority. But it is constantly present, as the work of Derek Morgan,[33] including his paper in this volume, amply illustrates. As elsewhere, ideology is cloaked by framing solutions as inevitable consequences of unquestioned and supposed unproblematic legal institutions such as the sanctity of contract and private property. But how well do these concepts fit, and what is the significance of trying to fit them, to the "sale" of a baby or rights over an embryo? How useful are notions of agency when the principal is mentally handicapped or comatose?

All the questions discussed in these papers are matters of ethics, they are about the decisions that we should take, about matters of right and wrong.[34] Should we permit involuntary sterilisation, is research upon embryos morally justifiable, of what moral significance is the "living will" of the terminally ill patient,[35] should we allow assisted reproduction and, if so, what limits should we put on the doctors, does negligence and therefore fault have a part to play in the medical setting? It would be idle to pretend that philosophers have the answers to these questions. They have answers and different philosophies, most obviously utilitarianism[36] and Kantianism,[37] the one concerned with a maximisation of welfare, the other with (in contemporary jargon) "taking rights seriously,"[38] have different answers. It would also be rash to ignore the political ideologies embraced by particular philosophies. Nor are philosophical statements necessarily always internally consistent. One of the more disappointing features of the Warnock report[39] is the incoherence of its philosophy, at times informed by utilitarian considerations, at other by deontological,[40] at times firmly wedded to autonomy, at others adopting a paternalistic or moralistic stance.[41] This leads it into the flabbiest of reasoning, as where it concludes that surrogacy (for the fertile) is "totally ethically unacceptable"[42] without telling us whose ethics have imposed this judgment or offering (for example) any appreciation of why some women might find the use of surrogates convenient. Instead it supports its objection by resort to classical Kantian argument (people should not "treat others as a means to their own ends"),[43] an argument curiously overlooked in its discussion of embryo experimentation, artificial insemination,[44] egg and embryo donation.

We can learn from the errors of the Warnock report. Whatever moral argument we use to support a particular policy must be coherent, it must be internally consistent, it must be justifiable to "significant others."[45] A series of inconclusive test matches has been played between proponents of different schools of philosophy. Neither side is ever likely to concede defeat. But out of the interminable wrangles does come a sharpened awareness of the issues, the problems and the concepts that are the tools of the argument. What's so special about rights?[46] What rights do we have? (Is there a "right to reproduce?") What does the maximisation of welfare entail? What does treating persons as equals involve? Does it include the right to equal treatment?[47] How important is autonomy? Does paternalism respect persons or can this be achieved only through recognition of individual autonomy?[48] What is a "person"? When does personhood begin and end? Can we satisfactorily distinguish between a pre-embryo (or conceptus), an embryo and a foetus?[49] And, if so, how? Do the unborn come into a utilitarian calculus? The questions are endless.[50]

What is important is that the debate has commenced. It will be enriched by dialogues such as those which took place at University College London in the autumn of 1987. It is to be hoped that a wider audience will profit from the reproduction of the papers given, and that fruitful debate on the many vital issues discussed in this collection will be thereby stimulated.

Notes

[1] Questions of law and medical ethics have been included in previous *Current Legal Problems*. An early example is I. Kennedy (1969) 22 C.L.P. 102. More recently see the articles in (1986) 39 *Current Legal Problems* by Mary Warnock and M.D.A. Freeman (pp. 17, 33 respectively).

[2] See P. Singer and D. Wells, *The Reproduction Revolution*, O.U.P. 1984.

[3] See *e.g.* Paul Johnson, *The Times*, August 26, 1985 (and correspondence in *The Times*, August 27, to September 2, 1985).

[4] On the compromise see V. Greenwood and J. Young, *Abortion in Demand*, Pluto Press, 1976. Two questions of which it has failed to provide answers are the "Morning-after" pill and the legality of inserting an I.U.D. after intercourse. There is a good discussion of these and other problems in M. Brazier, *Medicine, Patients and the Law*, Penguin, 1987, Chap. 12.

[5] Prompted by the Baby Cotton Affair (see *Re C.* [1985] F.L.R. 846). See C. Dyer, "Baby Cotton and the Birth of a Moral Panic," *The Guardian*, January 15, 1985 and A. Hutchinson and D. Morgan, "A Bill Born from Panic," *The Guardian*, July 12, 1985.

[6] Including a large number of attempts to amend abortion legislation and most notably Enoch Powell's Unborn Children (Protection) Bill in 1985.

[7] D.H.S.S., *Human Fertilisation and Embryology: A Framework for Legislation*, Cm. 259. (1987).

[8] [1986] A.C. 112.

[9] See Second Report of Voluntary Licensing Authority for Human *In Vitro* Fertilisation and Embryology, 1987, p. 8 and Annex 1.

[10] *Op. cit.* note 7.

[11] *Cf.* B. Hoggett's paper (at p. 95). See also A. Grubb and D. Pearl, "Sterilisation and the Courts," (1987) C.L.J. 439.

[12] Mental Health Act 1959. This was amended in 1982. The law now is contained in the Mental Health Act 1983.

[13] Prompted initially by the case of Jeanette (*Re B.* [1987] 2 All E.R. 206) and coming to the fore in three cases, of which subst. in 13 *T.* v. *T.* [1988] 2 W.L.R. 189 is the most fully reported.

[14] M.D.A. Freeman, *post*, p. 55: B. Hoggett, *post*, p. 85.

[15] But see the way Latey J. circumvented this in *Re Adoption Application* 212/86, [1987] 2 F.L.R. 291

[16] Readers will, I am sure, pardon the incorrect French: *en ventre son réfrigérateur* does not sound as good!

[17] In *Pettitt* v. *Pettitt* [1970] A.C. 777. See also Lord Reid, "The Judge as Law Maker" 12 J.S.P.T.L. 22.

[18] Most memorably in its report on *Divorce* (Cmnd. 3123, 1966). See also its Working Paper on *Illegitimacy* (Working Paper No. 74, 1979).

[19] Another advocate (Simon Lee) calls it a "Super-Warnock" (see "Re-reading Warnock" in *Rights and Wrongs in Medicine*, King Edward's Hospital Fund for London, (P. Byrne, ed.) 1986, pp. 37–52 at 48).

[20] *Report of the Inquiry into the Care and Supervision provided in relation to Maria Colwell (the Field-Fisher report)* H.M.S.O. 1974.

[21] *A Child in Mind*, L.B. of Greenwich, 1987.

[22] *Whose Child?*, L.B. of Lambeth, 1987.

[23] The publication in 1987 of a new journal *Bioethics* (by Blackwells) brings this home. It is to contain reports on recent developments in bioethics in several different countries (see vol. 1(2) at pp. iii–iv).

[24] See *Bioethics*, vol. 1, pp. 163–174 (1987) for an English translation of the *Final Report of the Netherlands State Commission on Euthanasia*, including the proposed amendments to the Criminal code. See also J.K.M. Gevers, "Legal Developments Concerning Active Euthanasia on Request in the Netherlands" *Bioethics*, vol. 1, pp. 136–162 (1987).

[25] See *post*, 150. See also the B.M.A. call for the introduction of no-fault liability insurance (*The Times*, May 15, 1987).

[26] (1986) 31 D.L.R. 1 (4th ed.) (and see *post*, 63, 66).

[27] *In the Matter of "Baby M"*, Superior Court of New Jersey, 217 N.J. Super. 313 (1987), reversed by New Jersey Supreme Court (1988) 14 F.L.R. 2007.

[28] *In re Quinlan* 355 2d 647 (1976).

[29] *Bouvia* v. *County of Riverside*. The Riverside Superior Court decision is conveniently found in Robert F. Weir (ed.), *Ethical Issues In Death and Dying* (2nd ed. 1986), Columbia Univ. Press, pp. 381–384. In 1986, an appellate court ruled unanimously that Elizabeth Bouvia, at the time a patient in another hospital, was entitled to have a nasogastric tube removed according to her wishes.

[30] *Bioethics*, vol. 1(3) is a Special Issue devoted to this subject. See also the QUALYS debate, as exemplified by J. Harris (1987) 13 J.Med.Ethics 117.

[31] *R.* v. *Ethical Committee of St. Mary's Hospital, ex parte Harriott*, *The Independent*, October 27, 1987.

[32] See, further, G. Calabresi and P. Babbitt, *Tragic Choices*, Norton, 1978.

[33] See "Making Motherhood Male" 11 J.S.L. (1984) and "Who To Be or Not To Be" (1985) 49 M.L.R. 358 (1986). Forthcoming is *The Moral Economy of Surrogacy*, Gower.

[34] As to which see J. Glover, *Causing Death and Saving Lives*, Penguin, 1977 and J. Mackie, *Ethics: Inventing Right and Wrong*, Penguin, 1977.

[35] See "The Right to Refuse Treatment: A Model Act," (1983) 73 Amer. J. of Public Health, 918–921 (also in Weir, *op. cit.*, note 29, pp. 194–204).

[36] See J. Smart and B. Williams, *Utilitarianism—For and Against*. Cambridge Univ. Press, 1973.

[37] T.L. Beauchamp and J.F. Childress, *Principles of Biomedical Ethics* (2nd ed. 1983), Chap. 3 is an excellent discussion in the context of medical ethics.

[38] See R. Dworkin, *Taking Rights Seriously* (revised ed., 1978), Duckworth. And, falling into the jargon, R. Adler, *Taking Juvenile Justice Seriously* (1985), Scottish Academic Press and M.D.A. Freeman, "Taking Children's Rights Seriously" *Children and Society*, Vol. 1(4) 1988, pp. 299–319.

[39] Cmnd. 9314 (1984): republished as Mary Warnock, *A Question of Life* Blackwell, 1985.

[40] *Cf.* Foreword, para. 4 (deontological) and para. 11.18 (utilitarian).

[41] See para. 8.10.

[42] See para. 8.17.

[43] *Idem.* The Kantian objection is that a person should *never* be treated *only* as a means.

[44] Though Andrea Dworkin is scathing in her criticism of those who see any analogy between A.I.D. and surrogacy (quoted in Corea, *The Mother Machine*, Women's Press, 1988, pp. 226–227). And see also her *Right-Wing Women*, 1983.

[45] *Cf.* H. Becker, *Outsiders*, Free Press, 1963, p. 9.

[46] A question asked puzzlingly in a valuable article by H. Bedau (See Social Philosophy and Policy vol. 1, no. 2 (1984)).

[47] *Cf.* R. Dworkin, *op. cit.*, note 38, pp. 227–228.

[48] *Cf.* J. Harris, *The Value of Life*, R.K.P. 1985, Chap. 10.

[49] See L. Fleming, "The Moral Status of the Foetus: A Reappraisal" *Bioethics* vol. 1, pp. 15–34 (1987); K. Dawson, "Segmentation and Moral Status in Vivo and in Vitro: A Scientific Perspective" *Bioethics*, vol. 2, pp. 1–14 (1988).

[50] The latest to hit the headlines is the moral legitimacy of using foetal tissue from aborted foetuses to treat persons with Parkinson's disease. See *The Sunday Times*, April 17, 1988. See further P. McCullagh, *The Foetus as Transplant Donor: Scientific, Social and Ethical Perspectives*, 1987.

Embryos' "Rights": Abortion and Research[1]

MARGARET BRAZIER

"If you ban research on embryos, you must rewrite the laws on abortion."[2] Thus Professor Robert Edwards concluded his case for permitting experiments on embryos in a public lecture at Manchester last spring. The proposition that no rational system of law can operate relatively liberal rules on abortion yet still prohibit research is one which unites the extreme camps in the debate on embryo research. Those who passionately oppose research as a violation of life probably do regard attempts to ban research as the thin end of the wedge which (they hope) may lead to repeal of the 1967 Abortion Act.[3] Opponents of liberal legislation permitting experimentation on embryos well beyond the 14 day limit proposed by Warnock[4] link abortion and research for two possible reasons.

The primary reason for linking issues of abortion and experimentation is grounded in the philosophical debate on the embryo and personhood. It is a debate which in our present society, with its diversity of religious and cultural perspectives, can provide no rational conclusion which will stand alone as the sole criterion for determining what may or may not be done to embryos *in vivo* or *in vitro*. A secondary reason may, perhaps, be tactical and political. A growing body of feminist opinion is disturbed by experimentation and the panoply of modern reproductive medicine. While ambivalent about the ethics of abortion[5] most feminists nevertheless remain "pro-choice" on that issue. Linking abortion and research may be seen as part of an attempt to regain feminist backing for research.

What I want to attempt to do in this paper is to establish that the relevant criteria on which legislation on abortion should be based are not identical to the criteria on which legislation on research should rationally be based. And, very tentatively, I try to outline criteria on which Parliament should approach the issue of research. The occasionally scathing criticism by ethicists of the

Warnock Committee's proposals has overlooked one crucial
question. When you are making laws on such ethical "hot
potatoes" there are two separate questions to be addressed. What
is the correct ethical stance in pure theory? On what ethical basis
can you then legislate to create effective and enforceable legal
rules?

In the title to this paper the word "rights" is deliberately placed
in quotation marks. It is trite now to repeat that the embryo as
such outside its mother, the embryo created in a Petrie dish, has
no legal rights.[6] It exists and dies in a legal limbo. For a common
lawyer, the starting point of any effort to establish what should be
the "rights" of embryos must be to review the existing law and
analyse what "rights," if any, existing law has accorded to the
embryo *in vivo*. The law presently recognises the unborn as having
status[7] in three main respects, for the purposes of succession, by
virtue of the Congenital Disabilities (Civil Liability) Act 1976 and
in the legislation on abortion and child destruction. None of these
three instances confers enforceable rights on the embryo before
birth nor do they accord to the embryo the full status of a "person
in being."

The right to inherit[8] and to be classified a dependant for the
purposes of the Fatal Accidents Act[9] enures to a child *en ventre sa
mère* at the date of the deceased's death; but crystallises only at
birth—live birth. It is at most a contingent right.

In England no definitive ruling at common law resolved whether
a child damaged before birth could sue in tort.[10] The 1976 Act[11]
creates at best (and pretty ineffectually) rights which are once
again contingent[12] and derivative. The disabled baby has a remedy
only when liability in tort to the affected parent is proved.[13] He
may not in general sue his mother[14] and the identification of
mother and child is strengthened further by the provision that any
contributory negligence on her part may result in a reduction of
the damages payable to the child.[15] The Act confers on a child
born alive a right to a healthy body but is as much concerned with
protecting parental rights to beget and conceive healthy offspring,
as any independent rights of the affected infant herself.

The policy behind the legislation criminalising abortion comes
closest to recognising independent rights of the embryo. But it is
questionable whether English law (even prior to the Abortion Act
1967) recognised a child before birth as enjoying the same status as
that same child moments after birth. Were the status of the
embryo to be equated with the status of the child, criminal
offences of abortion and child destruction would be unnecessary.
The killing of the "child" would in all cases logically constitute the

offence of murder. The complex, if ancient, case-law on when the baby attains life independent of its mother would be otiose.[16] Blackstone affirmed,

> "Life is an immediate gift from God, a right inherent by nature in every individual, and it begins in contemplation of the law as soon as an infant is able to stir in the mother's womb."[17]

This has never represented the reality of the common law. Murder requires the unlawful killing of " . . . a reasonable creature *in rerum natura* under the King's peace."[18] At common law the killing of the child in the womb constituted a misdemeanour (not a felony) and that only once the child had quickened in the womb. Now the latter condition (abolished in 1837) can be dismissed as indicating a lack of understanding of the development of embryos, but taken together the common law gives us a number of guidelines on the limits of legal protection of embryos. The condition that no crime was committed until quickening derived in large part from theological opinion that ensoulment took place only at quickening. Yet the classification of abortion as a lesser offence than murder indicates that the common law accorded a lesser status to life before birth even after quickening and presumed ensoulment.

Coke's classic definition of murder limits that offence to "a reasonable creature . . . under the King's peace." That latter phrase in practice excluded only outlaws and the King's enemies in time of war from the ambit of the crime of murder. But it does act as a key to the primary function of the criminal law, to preserve order.[19] The deliberate destruction of the embryo in the womb may be as sinful as the slaughter of a newborn child or an adult. The commission of a moral wrong was, at least at common law, a pre-requisite of categorising an act as a crime. But where the embryo's destruction is encompassed by the mother's wish, and should it be against her will a crime is committed against her, then the threat of disorder resulting from the embryo's "death" is minimal. No chain of revenge and retaliation is set in motion.

Legislation from 1837 to 1967 considerably elaborated and extended the scope of the criminal law on abortion and child destruction. Does that legislation evidence a fundamental change of policy on embryos' rights? The 1967 Act itself must be left out of consideration because the debate on embryos' rights questions the grounds on which that Act is founded. The continuing controversy over the Abortion Act all too often overlooks the

remarkable extent to which the judgment in *R.* v. *Bourne*[20] held
that the Offences against the Person Act 1861[21] operated a much
less than total ban on abortion. Directing the jury in Dr. Alec
Bourne's trial for performing an abortion on a young girl who had
been brutally raped, Macnaghten J. found that as procuring miscarriage was an offence only when unlawfully attempted, the statute
recognised that such an operation might under certain conditions be
lawfully performed. Where a woman's life or health were at risk,
where "the probable consequence of the continuance of the pregnancy will be to make the woman a physical or mental wreck"[22]
abortion might lawfully be carried out. A doctor who failed to
operate to save the life of a woman by performing an abortion might
himself be in "grave peril" of facing prosecution for
manslaughter.[23]

Well before 1967 the law, while recognising the *status* of the
embryo, afforded it *rights* subordinate to its mother's right to life
and health. The foundation of laws in England on abortion rests on
the inevitable conflict between the interests of the embryo and those
of its mother. The 1967 Act, or more relevantly the interpretation of
that Act by many doctors, has altered and extended the definition of
the mother's rights but not the fundamental policy of the law to
subordinate any rights the embryo may have to those of his
mother.[24] The embryo has a recognised status worthy of legal
protection but not at the mother's expense.

No such conflict of interests affects the issue of research on
embryos. The status accorded to the embryo *in vivo* must rationally
be accorded to the embryo *in vitro*.[25] No other individual's rights or
autonomy are violated by offering absolute protection to that
embryo from destruction or interference other than for the
embryo's own benefit.

Tracing the development of the current policy underlying English
law and abortion reveals a policy which permits abortion on
grounds which do not necessarily require legitimation of research.
But is the policy sustainable on grounds other than its historical
evolution? This question requires consideration of whether the law
ought in 1988 to afford any status to the embryo, and if it ought,
whether the rights arising from that status can properly be subordin-
ated to the mother's rights.

To determine whether any status should be accorded to the
embryo requires examination of the ethical debate on embryos
as persons. That embryos are not persons in being for the purposes of the law but are recognised as enjoying a status deserving of protection must be justified. Embryos may not enjoy
rights but duties are owed to them. Is this compromise rationally

sustainable? Four schools of thought are current. (1) Embryos command moral respect as human reproductive products.[26] (2) At the moment of fertilisation when the sperm and ovum unite a unique individual is created with its own unique genetic pattern. That individual is arguably from that point on as entitled to respect as you or me.[27] Both these arguments demand that embryos be afforded status from fertilisation.[28] The arguments to the contrary deny any specific status to humanity as such. Respect for human reproductive products on those grounds alone is "speciesist."[29] What entitles you and me to ethical status over and above that of my new puppy is our human "personhood." But on this issue the two schools of thought whose reasoning would deny all embryos rights disagree. The third argument in the debate contends that just as *brain death* is now generally accepted as marking the ending of life so *brain life* marks the beginning of personhood.[30] When the embryo begins to develop those parts of the brain which will eventually endow it with a sense of human identity it acquires status as a person at about ten weeks into pregnancy.[31] The final, and more extreme, argument demands that a being have an actual capacity for self awareness and an ability to value its individual existence before it acquires status as a person. On that reasoning, personhood is not acquired until some considerable period after birth.[32]

It is a debate incapable of resolution in a form which could provide definitive legal criteria on which to base laws on either abortion or research. For the chasm which separates the participants is unbridgeable. For those who believe that human life has divine origins and accept at least the proposition that human beings *may* possess as well as this material body an immaterial and immortal soul it follows that they are necessarily "speciesist." Human life is different, is superior in status to animal life. We may not know (and I suspect can never know) when and how that soul enters the embryo. But as it arguably happens as the genetic pattern of the individual is set, then, from that moment on that organism has a status worthy of respect. Now those ethicists who deny humanity status simply as humanity (in general and with certain notable exceptions)[33] do not accept or believe in the concept of ensoulment. However, just as I cannot prove that the soul exists so they cannot prove that it does not. We reach stalemate.

An individual woman who believes (as I do) on religious or other grounds that human life as such, the human organism, commands respect necessarily must accept that an embryo within her enjoys a status equal to her own.[34] But as perception of that

14   *Embryos' "Rights": Abortion and Research*

status derives from the presence or absence of belief in the unique nature of humanity, and the veracity or otherwise of that belief can never be established by tangible objective criteria, no one has a right in a democratic society to compel another woman to regulate her life, and curtail her freedom, on the basis of a belief that she does not share.

The inherent problem for someone who holds such a view is this. Once one accepts the embryo as having status as a human person, how can you in the next breath allow that that human may be destroyed. After all were there to be a substantial body of opinion that persons with red hair were not human but descended from the devil, that would not persuade me to say that it was therefore permissible for those genuinely holding those beliefs to kill all redheads.

The examples are distinguishable first, because of the inability to prove the humanity of the embryos, and secondly, because the context of abortion is unique. It is not simply a case of A killing B even when B is recognised as a human person. As Judith Jarvis Thomson[35] eloquently argues, the issue is not, should the mother be prevented from destroying the embryo, but shall the law compel her to sustain its life and growth for the nine months from fertilisation to birth? For the lawyer in addition to these arguments which distinguish abortion with its concomitant conflict of interests from embryo research, there is the further question of the enforceability of restrictive abortion laws and whether the other evils that would flow from a restrictive regime would outweigh any arguable benefits. Women from countries which restrict abortion come to England now. Several still die, or irretrievably prejudice their health. English women with money, if we restrict abortion, will go abroad. Others will resort to the backstreets. The embryo's "right to life" will not be significantly enhanced. Women's lives may be forfeit.[36]

Of the criteria applicable to determine legal rules on abortion only one remains centrally relevant to the debate on experimentation on embryos. And that is the status which should be accorded to the embryo which, I have argued, is a circular debate. The central thesis of whether or not humanity is simply a rational animal whose rationality alone commands respect or a unique, divinely created species is unprovable either way.[37] It is essential therefore to examine the consequences of the disputed status of the embryo and to search for further criteria unrelated to the status of the embryo on which to found legislation regulating research.

The consequence of the disputed status of the embryo in the context of abortion is that the proponents of the view that the embryo is as fully human as you or I cannot force that view on women who reject it. It does not follow that the disputed status of the embryo concurrently legitimates research by persons rejecting that view of humanity. The "not proven" status of the embryo gives rise rather to a strong presumption that it be not interfered with where no other person's rights are in issue.[38] Consider this example. Explosives have been set the day before to detonate and destroy a crumbling factory and its chimneys. Those who will detonate the explosion are a mile away from the site. Ten minutes before the agreed time, an onlooker says that he saw a tramp climbing through all the defences and into the factory. None of the security men employed to guard the site at night saw him. The evidence for a human being within the factory is thin. Yet it would be both illegal and unethical to go ahead with the plan to detonate the factory.

The trouble with the embryo is that whereas men can be sent in to search for the hypothetical tramp, we can not resolve the disputed nature of the embryo. That is frustrating and inconvenient, particularly for scientists who see great potential benefit in mankind in general from freedom to pursue research. Therefore as the contention that the embryo is fully human does not command universal support, the disputed nature of the embryo cannot for Parliament conclude the debate.

Other criteria by which to judge whether or not to permit research must be sought, but the burden of proof lies on the proponents of research. That is the consequence of the not proven nature of the embryo. The potential benefits of research have been well rehearsed and fall into four main categories (1) improvement in techniques to alleviate infertility, particularly *in vitro* fertilisation, (2) the development of improved means of contraception, (3) detection at an early stage of genetic defects offering greater opportunities to eradicate genetic disease, and (4) the potential for the use of early embryonic tissue or even organs to transplant into sick adults and children.[39] One example given is the use of foetal tissue in the treatment of Alzheimer's Disease.

The realistic likelihood of research on embryos resulting in the postulated benefits is itself hotly disputed.[40] The scientific debate is not one into which a lawyer can fully enter. The current White Paper[41] on Human Fertilisation and Embryology presents members of Parliament with two options. The first will permit research by clinics licensed by the Statutory Licensing Authority but only in the first 14 days subsequent to fertilisation. The second would prohibit any research unrelated to the re-implantation of a specific embryo or embryos in the womb. The Government's present proposals exclude any experimentation beyond 14 days and any such research in fact conducted would constitute a criminal offence. Members of Parliament will be given a free vote as the Government consider the issue to be one for individual Members to consult and follow their conscience.

Evaluation of the scientific data should be Parliament's first task. The disputed claims on the benefits of research must be investigated. In particular the extent to which the benefits claimed for research are attainable within a 14 day period must be closely scrutinised. The more vociferous proponents of research have pressed for a 28–42 day limit. It may be that attempts will be made to amend the Government Bill to extend the permissible research period. Before endorsing any 14 day limit Parliament should ensure that the consequent violation of what may be a human being is justified by the ensuing advantages to humanity as a whole. The selection of 14 days has to be recognised as a compromise.[42] It would be unfortunate if it proved to be a compromise with which nobody was comfortable.

Next Parliament must address the ethics of research if Members are satisfied that the preponderance of scientific opinion suggest that ascertainable benefits are attainable within the 14 days limit proposed or some longer timespan commanding majority support in the House. The nature of the benefits likely to be derived from research must (a) be evaluated in themselves and (b) weighed against any detriments.

Opinion polls on embryo research indicate unsurprisingly that a majority of those polled favour research which may lead to the eradication of genetic disease. The benefit to families haunted by congenital disease is very obvious and emotionally powerful. At present however what is envisaged is not that research offers a prospect of "curing" a "defective" embryo, but that more effective means of diagnosis may be developed to detect and destroy the "defective" embryo.[43] On that hypothesis the perceived benefit of the research proposed can have little weight for those whose perception of the nature of the embryo is as fully human from fertilisation onwards. The procedure cannot be justified as sacrificing the few to save the many. It becomes sacrificing the few to learn how to sacrifice the many.[44]

Improved techniques to alleviate infertility would clearly benefit those many couples who now suffer grievous disappointment. IVF is at present a notably unsuccessful treatment.[45] But before accepting that benefit without question two significant issues must be addressed. (1) Can we afford IVF within the present National Health Service? To improve the technique without realistic prospect of it being available to the majority of couples would be a lamentable policy. (2) Should we before concentrating such effort and resources on the symptoms of infertility address much greater effort to its causes and prevention?

The benefits claimed for research must be scrutinised with care. They should not be accepted as dogma. What of the detriments? Are there any save for those who share my perception of the embryo's status? There are two. General unease and revulsion against the notion of experimentation is expressed by numbers of people who have no reasoned or informed opinion on the nature of the embryo. And a tide of informed feminist opinion is running against research.

A great deal of elegant and eloquent prose has been written to condemn the view that people's instinctive feelings have relevance in assessing the ethics of embryo research. Baroness Warnock[46] in particular has received a great deal of, largely unjustified, criticism. The argument that subjective feelings are ethically irrelevant goes thus. As R.M. Hare[47] puts it:

> "It will not do just to take the existence of a widespread feeling that the experiments are wrong as somehow proving that they *are* wrong. There is a widespread feeling in Iran that women ought to have an inferior status to men, and in South Africa that blacks ought to be subordinate to whites."

Quite obviously both those latter propositions appall me. But Hare stands Lady Warnock's arguments about taking account of instinctive feelings on their head. Of course people reacting "Ugh" to the thought of embryo experiments does not *prove* that they are wrong. But it is relevant to how Parliament acts on the issue. Legislation should command general support. Our legislators are representatives not delegates. Moral imperatives may often require that Parliament takes the lead in changing a climate of opinion, as was the case with capital punishment. But it is elitist in the extreme to dismiss the opinion of each and every citizen who cannot argue his case like a trained philosopher. Nor can it be so readily assumed that instinctive feelings have no purposive basis. The instinct to protect the young of the species even well before birth is essential to the continuation of that species.

The dismissal of feelings which are not informed in the philosopher's sense is perhaps part too of a historical tradition which dismisses emotion as a relevant factor in debate. Yet emotion is invoked in one specific sense by all the proponents of the case for experimentation. The tragedy of infertility is quite obviously the motivating factor in the work of Edwards and Steptoe and their colleagues. The care and concern they display to the women in their care is a credit to their profession. So one would expect perhaps that women above all would back research which *inter alia* promises greater relief of infertility. Why are a number of feminists now less than enthusiastic about embryo research and indeed many modern developments in reproductive medicine?

The focus in the debate on research has assumed without reasonable argument that women's rights and women's interests are enhanced by such developments. Robyn Rowland from Deakin University in Australia cast doubt on that proposition in the second volume of *Bioethics* this spring.[48] She highlighted the general invisibility of women in the debate, selecting a telling phrase from an Australian Senate report in which the women to whom embryos were returned were described not as women or mothers but "receptive uterine environments."

Two of the concerns of women in relation to embryo research centre around the effect of research and the technology which it is hoped will result from that research and women's autonomy. First, how are embryos to be created for research? If we opt for use of spare embryos there is consensus that their use must be with the couple's consent. Should we create specific research embryos the greater intrusion needed to collect ova as opposed to sperm means that women already scheduled for some sort of gynaecological intervention will be asked to "donate" ova. So in both scenarios the woman is already a patient. Is she truly free to make her own choice? If research embryos are to be specifically created drugs will have to be given to induce supra-ovulation. A woman will be subjected to a procedure unnecessary for the treatment of the condition for which she sought medical help.

Secondly, if technology resulting from research attains the desired benefits, say in the field of genetic disease, is there a risk that choice whether or not to use that technology would be restricted? This nearly happened with abortion. In *Emeh* v. *Kensington A.H.A.*[49] at first instance Park J. refused Mrs Emeh damages for the cost of bringing up her unplanned child subsequent to an admittedly negligent sterilisation. He held that her unreasonable refusal of a termination of the pregnancy constituted a *novus actus interveniens* making her solely responsible for the baby's birth. Fortunately the Court of Appeal overruled him.[50] But would a mother refusing IVF and screening of the embryo be at risk of an action for "wrongful life" from her child in certain jurisdictions.[51] Who would define groups "at risk" whom it might be contended should opt for IVF[52] and embryo screening? Am I, at 37, in such a group and therefore to be pressured into "high-tech" conception as well as "high-tech" birth?

I have addressed only some of the arguments advanced in the debate on embryos' "rights" and experimentation. I have deliberately omitted the "slippery slope" debate, regarding that as a slope on which I am the most likely person to slip. My central theme has been that it is for proponents of research to make their case, and to doubt the validity of certain of the benefits claimed for research. In equity opponents of research must too address and Parliament deliberate one very obvious consequence of a ban on research. The hoped for improvement in IVF must be sacrificed, and more critically the present procedure will necessarily be rendered less successful. For Parliament cannot rationally prohibit experimentation and permit the creation of several spare embryos to offer the best possible prospect of pregnancy with the consequence that a number of embryos must be destroyed either instantly or after freezing and having proved to be surplus to need. Destruction of the embryo cannot be preferable to research.[53]

Prohibition of the creation of spare embryos alone however will continue to leave certain embryos vulnerable. What should result where only one or two embryos are created but examination reveals that the embryo is defective. For a doctor to implant in the mother a defective embryo would be unethical. Therefore defective embryos will have to be destroyed. For myself I can just, despite my own perception of the embryo as fully human, reconcile the inevitable destruction of some embryos on analogy with abortion. The mother's right to refuse re-implantation of a defective embryo equates with her right to termination of pregnancy in cases of foetal handicap. Any different analysis would require the conclusion that *in vitro* fertilisation should itself be prohibited.[54] The present Government has entrusted Parliament with the ultimate responsibility for whether or not embryo research continues. The decision will rest with the conscience of each of our elected representatives. What Members of Parliament must decide is whether the destruction of what may be human beings can be permitted for the greater good of society as a whole. And they must be convinced that the goods claimed for such research is soundly based and not matched by equal detriments. The problems posed by the extent to which abortion law subordinates the embryo's rights to the mother's, and derogates from those rights to enhance those of the mother whom all accept as human, should not affect a judgment on research.

Notes

[1] For convenience alone and acknowledging the imprecision of the term I use the word 'embryo' throughout the paper to refer to all stages of development from zygote to the about to be born infant. I apologise for any infelicity or inaccuracy.

[2] "Experiments on Embryos: The Case For." Lecture delivered to the Centre for Social Ethics and Policy, University of Manchester in February 1987 to be published by Routledge in 1988. And see J.M. Harris *The Value of Life* at p. 117. "Nor can it be morally preferable to end the life of an embryo *in vivo* than it is to do so *in vitro*."

[3] The supporters of the Alton Bill to ban abortions after 18 weeks in general make no secret of their determination to outlaw abortion entirely in the long term.

[4] *Report of the Committee of Inquiry into Human Fertilisation and Embryology* Cmnd. 9314 (1984) The White Paper on *Human Fertilisation and Embryology: A Framework for Legislation* Cm. 259 November 1987 offers Parliament the options of a ban on experimentation or licensed research up to 14 days.

[5] See, for example, Linda Bird Francke *The Ambivalence of Abortion*; Allen Lane (1979).

[6] The Offences against the Person Act 1861 prohibits procuring miscarriage. An embryo *in vitro* is never carried by a woman and therefore, by chance and the outdated nature of the criminal law, and not by virtue of any policy judgment, it falls outside the law's ambit.

[7] I use the term "status" to indicate that the common law and statute recognised the existence of the embryo while leaving open the question of what rights the embryo enjoyed or what duties were owed to the embryo. It is not a term of art.

[8] Administration of Estates Act 1925 s.55(2); see generally *Williams on Wills* (5th ed.) Chap. 73.

[9] *The George and Richard* (1871) LR 3 A. & E. 466.

[10] The existence of a duty to an unborn child at common law was conceded in *Williams* v. *Luff, The Times*, February 14, 1978, and see *McKay* v. *Essex A.H.A.* [1982] Q.B. 1166.

[11] The Act was based on proposals from the Law Commission; Law Com. No. 60 (1974) "Injuries to Unborn Children." And see P.J. Pace "Civil Liability for Pre-Natal Injuries" (1977) 40 M.L.R. 141; K.M. Stanton (1976) 6 Fam. Law 206; P.J. Cane (1977) 51 A.L.J. 704.

[12] The child must be born alive; s.1(1).

[13] See s.1(3).

[14] Section 1(1) provides that any person "other than the child's own mother" may be answerable under the Act for an occurrence as a result of which the child suffers disabilities. In any case, as liability under the Act depends on liability in tort to the "affected parent" mothers could only have been made liable were they held to owe a duty in tort to their child's father not to damage the child *in utero*. Section 2 of the Act provides a single exception to the general maternal immunity

> "A woman driving a motor vehicle when she knows (or ought reasonably to know) herself to be pregnant is to be regarded as being under the same duty of care for the safety of her unborn child as the law imposes on her with respect to the safety of other people; and if in consequence of her breach of that duty her child is born with disabilities which would not otherwise have

been present, those disabilities are to be regarded as damage resulting from her wrongful act and actionable accordingly at the suit of the child."

section 2 thus furnishes a rare instance of a legal duty owed directly to the unborn infant.

[15] s.1(7).

[16] *R. v. Brain* (1834) 6 C. & P. 350; *R. v. Reeves* (1839) 9 C. & P. 25 and see S.B. Atkinson (1904) 20 L.Q.R. 134.

[17] See *Commentaries* (15th ed.) Vol. 1 at p. 129 and see Pace *op. cit.* at p. 141.

[18] Coke 3 Inst. 47; and see Smith & Hogan *Criminal Law* (5th ed.) pp. 273–278.

[19] See, for example, Edmund-Davies J. addressing the Magistrates Association (1963) 19 *The Magistrate* 183.

[20] [1939] 1 K.B. 687; and see *R. v. Newton and Stungo* [1958] Crim.L.R. 469; Havard "Therapeutic Abortion" [1958] Crim.L.R. 600.

[21] ss.58–59; and see the Infant Life (Preservation) Act 1929.

[22] At p. 694.

[23] At p. 693.

[24] On the detailed workings of the Abortion Act 1967 see A.J.C. Hoggett "The Abortion Act 1967" [1968] Crim.L.R. 247; J.M. Finnis [1971] Crim.L.R. 3.

[25] As J.M. Harris *op. cit.* at p. 117 maintains but omits to highlight the crucial distinction that the rights of the embryo *in vivo* may be in conflict with the mother's rights.

[26] As Ian Kennedy has argued; see *The Times*, June 8, 1984.

[27] See the minority dissent in the Warnock Report at pp. 91–93. And see Teresa Inglesias "In Vitro Fertilisation, The Major Issues" (1984) 10 J. Med. Ethics 32; Oliver O'Donovan, *Begotten or Made* O.U.P. 1984.

[28] The second argument runs into some problems from the intrinsic nature of the fertilisation process. There is no single definable moment when the gametes fuse. Presumably the nature of the argument requires that respect for the embryo dates from the moment of its inception. The first argument that human reproductive products deserve respect *per se* avoids this conundrum. But does it require a ban on experimentation on sperm and ova?

[29] See J.M. Harris *op. cit.* at p. 23.

[30] See M. Lockwood "When does a life begin?" in *Moral Dilemmas in Medicine* ed. M. Lockwood (1985).

[31] See Keith Ward "Persons, Kinds and Capacities" in *Rights and Wrongs in Medicine* at p. 53 (King's College Studies (1985–6)).

[32] See J.M. Harris *op. cit.* at pp. 18–25 and Chaps. 10 and 11. And see Jonathan Glover *Causing Death and Saving Lives*, Pelican (1977).

[33] See Ward op. cit. and see G.R. Dunstan "The Moral Status of the Human Embryo: A Tradition Recalled" (1984) 10 J. Med. Ethics 38. Ward and Dunstan argue eloquently that the human soul is linked to the human brain and invoke too the tradition of the Church fathers conclude that ensoulment is likely to be concurrent with the beginnings of brain life.

[34] And therefore she cannot ethically terminate its existence. Neither the fact that the child was conceived as the result of rape nor that it was grossly deformed *ought* to justify the destruction of a child recognised by his mother as "fully human." But can/should the law even in a hypothetical society concurring in this perception of the sanctity of life enforce the attainment of the "ideal?" Should the mother not be left to decide the issue according to her conscience? Her sin (if any) is a matter between her and God.

[35] "A Defence of Abortion" in *The Philosophy of Law* at p. 112, ed. R.M. Dworkin (1977). But see the reply by J.M. Finnis "The Rights and Wrongs of Abortion" *op. cit.* at p. 129.

36 The statistics on the extent of illegal abortion and maternal mortality are unsurprisingly themselves much disputed see M. Simms [1970] Crim.L.R. 567, [1971] Crim.L.R. 86; J.M. Finnis [1971] Crim.L.R. 3.
37 As is the contention by Christian theologians that ensoulment takes place only at a much later stage than fertilisation. See the writings of Ward and Dunstan above at note 33.
38 For if the embryo is arguably human then it arguably acquires a right to autonomy which should not be violated unless protection of the embryo's rights violates the rights of beings who are indubitably human persons.
39 See R.G. Edwards "Experiments on Embryos: The Case For," above at note 2. Use of foetal tissue from aborted foetuses raises quite separate ethical issues.
40 See, for example, M. Rayner "Experiments on embryos; stick to the facts"; (1986) *New Scientist,* 27 February, 1986.
41 Cmd. 259 (1987).
42 The selection of a 14 day limit by the Warnock Committee endorsed in the White Paper is justified on the following grounds. 14 days marks the emergence of the "primitive streak" and the latest stage at which the fertilised ovum can divide to become identical twins. It is also the stage at which it can be discovered whether the organism will develop as an embryo or take a different course becoming for example a hydatiform mole.
43 And would the proposed ban on gene manipulation in the White Paper in any case outlaw such research? It is aimed at genetic engineering of humans with pre-determined characteristics but the wording of the Bill will need careful scrutiny.
44 The ethics of whether an individual may ever be sacrificed for the good of society have been little explored in the debate on embryo research. Christian tradition recognised such a principle within the context of the "just war." The use of foetal tissue from live embryos *in vitro* (as opposed to tissue taken from aborted embryos) might be seen in this light. But could the violation of X to benefit Y ever be justifiable?
45 15 per cent. Annex A: White Paper: 11.5 per cent. an average: *Report of the Voluntary Licensing Authority* (1986).
46 See "Do Human Cells Have Rights," Vol. 1 *Bioethics* 1 (1987).
47 "An Ambiguity in Warnock," Vol. 1 *Bioethics* 175 at p. 178 (1987).
48 "Making Women Visible in the Embryo Experimentation Debate," Vol. 1 *Bioethics* 179 (1987). And S. Uniacke "In Vitro Fertilisation and the Right to Reproduce," Vol. 1 *Bioethics* 241 (1987).
49 *The Times,* January 3, 1983.
50 [1984] 3 All E.R. 1099 C.A. But the judgment of Waller L.J. is open to the interpretation that refusal of lawful abortion in the first 12 weeks of pregnancy might have deprived Mrs Emeh of her remedy; see M. Brazier, *Medicine Patients and the Law,* Pelican (1987) at pp. 167–168.
51 For the present the judgment in *McKay* v. *Essex A.H.A.* [1982] Q.B. 1166 excludes such actions in England.
52 Screening might alternatively be carried out via natural conception *in vivo* and subsequent *lavage.* The objection that once routine such procedures might become "compulsory" remains the same.
53 See Simon Lee "Re-reading Warnock," in *Rights and Wrongs in Medicine* at p. 52.
54 Freezing of embryos, which the White Paper would permit, is problematical too. If "unwanted" the embryos will be destroyed.

Technology and the Political Economy of Reproduction

DEREK MORGAN

"...we lack a perspective for judgement of transformations that go so deep.... Everything around us is new and different—our concerns, our working habits, our relations with one another. Our very psychology has been shaken to its foundations, to its most secret recesses. Our notions of separation, absence, distance, return, are reflections of a new set of realities, though the words themselves remain unchanged. To grasp the meaning of the world of today we use a language created to express the world of yesterday."[1]

The contemporary debate concerning reproductive technologies and their impact on questions of sexuality takes place within a reawakening of recognition of the family as a politicised institution. A conservative notion of "family"—and of *the* family—is implicit in much recent social policy and explicit in the policing of sexuality.[2] For supporters of the family no new form of family is possible and for opponents of the legally defined family, namely marriage, only new forms of household are possible.[3] Conservative Government policy, meanwhile, rests on the Trinity of the Family, the Private Market and The Voluntary Sector.[4] Hence, its attempts in the last five years to enlarge both privately born responsibility and apparent private freedom from state structures, and its concern to constrain patterns of sexuality and reproduction because of the Family's supposed success in carrying out the tasks expected of it, evidencing a subtle redrawing or re-emphasising of the boundaries between the public and the private.[5]

It is important immediately to clarify the use of some familiar terms.

"The problem with using the terms "Left" and "Right" in this context relate to their traditionally being used to refer to political positions held on *public* affairs. Issues of sexual

23

morality, however, cross the boundaries of public and private. . . . Although the Moral Right's adherents are likely to be Conservative supporters, this cannot be assumed. The British moral lobby is politically non-aligned and thus cannot unproblematically be defined as part of the new Right, let alone of Thatcherism. That being said, the Moral Right's call for restoration of traditional morality, discipline and order coalesces neatly with Thatcher's call for a return to "Victorian" values . . . the Moral Right claims to speak for a silent, family-loving majority."[6]

One particular aspect of the desire to strengthen traditional family morality is to keep sex fundamentally concerned with parenthood and the need to preserve "natural" family relationships. In this way, the Conservative Government has given emphasis to the claims of the Moral Right, and has used its power to appropriate, maintain and control the ideologies of sexuality and gender produced and reproduced within various discourses to privilege those congenial to the Moral Right within official policy and practice.[7] These shifts have produced a new reliance on morality as a means of political mobilisation.[8] Assisted reproduction, which has the power not merely further to separate sex from reproduction, but also to separate biological from social parenthood, itself adds to the politicisation of family life and to what Alan Hunt has called the *familisation* of political life.[9] The interconnection between these realms is an important one to identify, because it serves to remind us that the familisation of political life tends to obscure that the private is "not natural but is itself a construction within a particular set of beliefs."[10] Nikolas Rose has suggested that this has at least four important consequences; it mystifies the fact that the state itself constructs the boundaries and limits of privacy; it legitimates the extent to which the state refuses to intervene into certain places or relations through its legal mechanisms; it masks the fact that privacy is all too often the right of men to dominate women and children, and it obscures the degree to which the state empowers welfare professionals to impose social norms on the family lives of certain sections of society, especially controlling women in their roles as wives and mothers.[11]

In parallel with this, Lorraine Harding has neatly encapsulated the dynamic of the relationship between law and social policy in her identification of the changing and emergent status of children, parents and parental substitutes as a major force in placing reproductive technologies firmly on the political and social agenda.[12] Her contention that uncertainty and conflict surrounding parental rights and responsibilities, the up-bringing, care and control of children conceived and born on the crest of the bio-technological tide, and the appropriate role of state agencies to oversee the developments of technology and the products of their conception, has established new questions. Who is eligible for reproductive assistance? On what conditions, and set by whom? What makes a good parent, in social and welfare terms?[13] This is mirrored by a reawakened concern about who can have access to relationships with children and for what reasons, a concern presaged by the rising rates of divorce and remarriage in Western societies and perceived needs to establish or maintain kin relationships in the face of the physical consequences of such separations.

Within these parameters, reproductive technology generates conflict. I want to suggest that it generates controversy of two particular and different sorts. Writing of *Gillick*,[14] Les Moran has suggested that the control of sexuality has been diversified through new technologies and the professions which have grown up to promote and attend upon them:

> "The particular issue raised in the case arises from the capacity of the medical regime to penetrate the 'private' space of the family and thereby supersede the familial regime of control. The hierarchical ordering of these domains of control is at the heart of the dispute."[15]

Mutatis mutandi reproductive technology. The report of the Ethics Committee of the Royal College of Obstetricians and Gynaecologists *In Vitro Fetilisation and Embryo Transfer*,[16] the Working Party of the Council for Science and Society[17] and the [*Warnock*] *Report of the Committee of Inquiry into Human Fertilisation and Embryology*[18] are just three from many examples of endorsements of *social* conditions which should pertain before the panoply of technological "assistance" can properly be contemplated. Artificial reproduction means that it is no longer necessary to determine reproduction according to who can have sex with whom, and the result is the construction of a matrix of hierarchies for determining who can have artificial reproduction with whom; AIH, AID, embryo transfer, and so on.[19] A form of technological incest—of "unnatural" relations—is thereby created to minimise the repugnance which might otherwise attach to some of manifold uses that technology, and to legitimate those "approved" forms of use and research.

But, as Edward Yoxen has forcefully reminded us, the language of nature is often used collusively and presumes or implies a shared agreement about common standards where none really exists; the symbolism of what nature permits is extremely powerful. According to Yoxen, science *is* the transformation of nature; we select bits of the external world and call them nature. We put together models of how we think the world is and of how we think it should be, a process which each culture does differently, and we call the resulting pictures "nature."[20] But cultural specificity recalls the kaleidoscopic nature of nature. Debate and discussion of reproductive technologies disclose fears which we harbour. These fears are present and revealed because the technologies question whether, when and with whom members of our species may reproduce; they stand to re-order much of our lives; "our sexual relations, our basic satisfactions, our kinship, our sense of meaning to life and what we have on our conscience."[21]

The second type of conflict which reproductive technologies generate is in the choices which they offer or mandate for individual women, and to a lesser extent men. This is echoed in the compromises which they suggest for the class woman, or man, and for different groups within those classes. In particular, as Ann Oakley has suggested, reproduction has come to be recognised as one area in which women are either liberated or oppressed, either free to determine and control their own individual and collective destinies or compelled to have them chosen and directed by others.[22] It is this, she argues, which underlines the dual nature of reproductive freedom; where *involuntary* reproduction can be eliminated and *involuntary* infertility overcome. Yet, while the state's intervention in political, social, economic and medical life continues to multiply, that control, so far as medicine is concerned, is exercised over the social and economic organisation of medical work, leaving the development and dispatch of technological innovation to the control of the profession.[23] The effect has been to create out of maternity a battlefield for not only patriarchal but professional supremacy;[24] "motherhood is a political battleground, a contested area for control—of women's bodies, of the fortunes of families, of the obligations of community support, of the constraints on choice."[25]

Reproductive technologies are not homogeneous in their presence, potential, impact or incidence. And this applies across potential user groups as well as across the different technologies.[26] For the moment it is sufficient to observe that reproductive technologies do not display many features of user friendliness which are claimed to mark out other artefacts of technological evolution. These two different types of conflict converge in a way which cautions an assessment and evaluation of reproductive technologies.

Family reform of the last one hundred years or so is a difficult area to chart, let alone navigate confidently.

> "The programmes of regulation of domestic, conjugal and reproductive arrangements, and the projects for reform of habitation, did not originate with 'the state.' Their initiators, supporters and allies were heterogeneous, the problems which they posed themselves were diverse. They were certainly bound up with systems of domination; if one takes this term in its sense of ruling or governing, shaping events to certain ends. But the ends they sought were not in any simple way functional to the state, to men or to the economy."[27]

This echoes clearly the view that women have not been passive victims or duped collaborators in these movements. Indeed, as with the reproductive technologies of the late twentieth century, they have often been active in campaigning for reform, for greater and more widely available access to provision, and have called upon the expertise of medical technologists, lawyers and social work professionals to back them up. That is an inversion of the way in which knowledge and expertise is frequently portrayed and used; it is a claim which will call for careful review and evaluation.

The Reprotechnologies: the Genesis of the Brave New World?

Aldous Huxley's book first published in 1932 has lent its title to critical assessments of disciplinary developments ranging from biology, physiology and psychology, through architecture, literature and cinema, to physics, chemistry and engineering. But it is with developments in biological sciences that the fashioning of the *Brave New World* has become most clearly identified. This is hardly surprising: Huxley's novel is a fabulous account of a world state in which social stability is assured by personal gratification and satisfaction based on a scientific caste system. It is reinforced by a sexual "freedom" which flows from the abandonment of family and the introduction of artificial reproduction which is controlled by the state; human beings are graded according to preplanned intelligence quotients, hatched in incubators and brought up in communal nurseries. The parallels between this foreboding model and some of the recent developments in reproductive technology are too close not to make the spectre of an alien and atomistic reproductive consciousness seem appropriate. The technological gradient appears to have become set towards the Utopia of which Huxley was fearful, rather than the community to which he aspired, one in which "science and technology would be used as though ... they had been made for man, not (as at present and still more so in the Brave New World) as though man were to be adapted and enslaved to them."[28]

A range of techniques can be identified within the broad penumbra of reproductive technology. It is, however, possible to divide these into so-called "old" and "new" categories.[29] Under the "old" listing would be found the cap, the sponge, the IUD, the sheath, and hormonal contraceptives. Abortion, sterilisation and vasectomy, complement mechanical procedures at birth, including episiotomies and Caesarian sections. "New" technologies encompass amniocentesis and the more recently developed chorionic villus sampling; foetal monitoring; pre-conception sex selection; post-conception sex determination; *in vitro* fertilisation, surrogacy, embryo transfer, egg donation, AID/H, embryo freezing, cloning and the development of an artificial placenta. The distinction between these categories is, however, challenged by Klein, who suggests that there is a pervasive link between all these different techniques, be they fashionably regarded as new or old.

> "As with the 'old' technologies the rule with the 'new' is that the less women interfere with the medical experts, the better.... There is no discussion about the social construction of motherhood and the question of real 'choice' a woman has in a society that continues to equate 'real' women with mother and wife."[30]

Some of these techniques are routinely established, either in what is euphemistically called animal husbandry or in human reproduction with what is characteristically known as a reasonable "success" rate. These would include sex determination and preselection. A second "group" might be thought of as experimental, in that their "success" rates are infrequent or low. Here, a common categorisation would encompass artificial insemination, *in vitro* fertilisation, and embryo transfer.

A third band of technologies are more futuristic and speculative, and involve the uses of cloning, parthenogenesis—the
production of an embryo from an egg without fertilisation by
sperm—and finally the development of an artificial placenta or
an artificial womb. For the purposes of this essay I want only
to review in any depth *in vitro* fertilisation and embryo transfer. This is not to suggest that the other technologies are unim-
portant, nor that those which figure as relatively long established technologies are unproblematic and do not illustrate
some of the thesis. Nor does it suggest that if we sort out our
thinking with reproductive technologies we will have made
major advances forward in the human condition and the eradication of unjust, prejudicial or barbaric actions and conditions.
It is, however, to argue that a study of reproductive technology
is important in thinking about who we are, and who we say we
want to become. In studying these developing techniques, an
examination of their practices may illuminate relationships and
responses which we take as established and for granted in a
new and challenging relief. As Michelle Stanworth proposes, a
study of reproductive technologies is appropriate because they
are controversial, and controversial "because they crystallise
issues at the heart of contemporary social and political strug-
gles over sexuality, reproduction, gender relations and the
family."[31]

In Vitro *Fertilisation and Embryo Donation*

This technique envisages the entry of male sperm into a woman's
egg outside her body. Fertilisation takes place in a petri dish—the
"test-tube" of popular imagery. The first external fertilisation is
noted in 1879, using a rabbit, with the first fertilisation of human
eggs occurring in 1968.[32] After fertilisation, the fertilised embryo is
reimplanted into the recipient's womb as the egg begins its process
of cell division. The "success" of the reimplantation is dependent
on the timing of the reimplantation and factors such as the quality of
the embryo, the fallopian tubes and the uterine environment. The
treatment of infertility through *in vitro* fertilisation has, and will
continue for the foreseeable future to have, a fairly low chance of
success; although in most *in vitro* fertilisation programmes there is a
direct relationship between multiple pregnancies and the number of
pre-embryos transferred. If one embryo is transferred, there is
about an 8 per cent. likelihood of pregnancy with two embryos, it
rises to 20 per cent. and with three transferred embryos, the success
rate is still only 30 per cent.[33] In most *in vitro* fertilisation

pregnancy; with two embryos, it rises to 20 per cent. and with three transferred embryos, the success rate is still only 30 per cent.[33] In most *in vitro* fertilisation programmes there is a direct relationship between the use of super ovulatory drugs and monozygotic twinning. At the Infertility Clinic, Hammersmith, statistics collected over the past eight years indicate that if three fertilisation attempts have failed, the chances of pregnancy on the fourth are lower than these previously quoted; only about 25 per cent. of embryo transfers result in pregnancy, and even if they implant, between 10 and 40 per cent. miscarry in the first few weeks of pregnancy. The process is time-consuming, emotionally and physically draining and is often advised only if there is "no satisfactory alternative."[34]

Women subjected to IVF are given hormones such as chlomiphene or pergonal to stimulate the production of more than one egg, or human chorionic gonadotropin, (HCG) to induce ovulation when the follicles containing the eggs are determined to have opened sufficiently. Eggs are removed at the optimum moment of the ovulatory process, which occurs at some stage over a four day period. Because of the individual nature of this process in different women, British reproductive physiologist Robert Edwards, who with Patrick Steptoe pioneered the technique of human *in vitro* fertilisation in the UK, once announced that "the day of the natural ovarian cycle is over."[35] That approach has now been superseded, however, by one which seeks to work with an individual woman's ovulatory cycle, and the increased use of cryopreservation of embryos, in order to decrease likely causes of technique failure. The major impediment to a higher "success" rate, which is claimed to stand at around 30 per cent. for the Bourn Hall Clinic,[36] is that IVF is presently considered as a last resort for the treatment of "infertility." The women who arrive at Bourn Hall for the commencement of IVF treatment have a mean age of 34–35. Edwards expresses his concern that they should be seen earlier and that IVF should be seen as a "treatment of first resort," even though the major type of infertility which they can treat successfully or overcome is male infertility—typically, males with immobile sperm or a low sperm count.[37] The "problem" of working with these types of infertility diagnosis is that men are notoriously coy about their admission of fertility deficiency, believing this in some way to reflect adversely on their sexuality and maleness.

More recently, scientists have developed what is known as the GIFT treatment, Gamete Infra-Fallopian Transfer. This involves mixing an egg or eggs from the ovaries with sperm and placing the eggs back into the recipient woman's fallopian tubes immediately, so that any resulting fertilisation takes places in the body. Some clinics have begun to report a higher success rate using this technique, and the first child born following its use in the United Kingdom was announced in 1987. One of the "problems" associated with this technique is recorded as being that "what happens to the [eggs and sperm] cannot be observed and recorded," meaning that it is not possible, as with *in vitro* fertilisation, to inspect the embryos for "abnormalities," which would commonly lead to them being "discarded rather than chance the risk of a defective baby."[38] Additionally, other experimental techniques at the early stages of development include Peritoneal Oocyte and Sperm Transfer (POST) and Vaginal Intra Peritoneal Sperm Transfer (VISPER), which have yet to report on established rates of successful delivery following use.

Following the successful birth of Britain's first "test tube" baby in July 1978, opposition within the medical establishment to *in vitro* fertilisation programmes weakened, and this type of "infertility treatment" is at January 1988 available in 30 centres licensed under the auspices of the professional self regulatory body, the Voluntary Licensing Authority. These centres are predominantly in London and other regional centres; there are presently no IVF centres in Wales or Northern Ireland, although Cardiff reports progress towards establishing the necessary medical personnel to make such a centre viable for the whole of the principality. Access to IVF treatment is thus dependent on " . . . a number of factors, including where patients live and the couples' financial resources."[39] Only one centre, in Manchester, is funded wholly by the NHS, the others have either a small recurrent budget of about £3,000 p.a., while most receive no funding.

"IVF clinics within the NHS make use of accommodation and certain facilities provided by the hospital but recurrent expenditure and most staff costs must be met with funding from outside sources. Some of these centres therefore ask patients for a specified donation for each treatment whilst others do not specify any particular sum and do not pressurise patients to pay. The major source of funding for IVF centres in the NHS sector is private practice. . . . Most IVF treatments in the UK are at present carried out in private clinics in return for fees."[40]

The *average* cost of IVF treatment at Bourn Hall, a private facility, is estimated to be about £10,000 per delivered baby, payable by the couple concerned. Four out of nearly 2000 births have produced serious "anomalies"; there being no apparent pattern to the deformities suffered. In Edwards' words, IVF is "merely assisting nature."[41]

Embryo Transfer and Embryo Research

Embryo transfer involves the placing of a fertilised egg of one woman into the uterus of another female. The parallels with animal husbandry, where again the technique was pioneered, have been drawn by a number of commentators. The Warnock Committee suggested approval of some limited form of embryo donation, in those cases where donated egg and semen were fertilised *in vitro*. They were opposed, however, to the form of such donation where the donor was inseminated with the semen of the genetic father and the fertilised egg washed out of the uterus through a lavage procedure before it had implanted in the uterine wall. This "embryo flushing" procedure has another possibility attached to it too; it could be developed and used for the genetic screening of chromosomal abnormalties. *Progress*, the pressure group formed to support research into reproductive issues has suggested that there are at least fifty types of severe congenital disease which may one day be detectable by pre-embryo screening, a direct spin off from IVF programmes.[42]

The perfection of "freezing" techniques means that frozen embryos (and latterly ova) can be stored for later use. This means that with the development of highly sophisticated surgical and monitoring techniques, the *genetic* mother need undergo only one operation for surgeons to recover several eggs, colloquially known as "harvesting."[43] She need then be reimplanted with only one, or at most two eggs at a time, thus avoiding the risks and complications of a multiple pregnancy. It is now possible to perform the reimplantations on a day-patient basis. Conversely, it is technically possible to use the techniques preferred by Professor Ian Craft at the Humana Wellington Hospital in London, of implanting multiple embryos and "selectively reducing" if any more than two or three successfully implant.[44]

Edwards has reported twenty "frozen" pregnancies. The conditions of storage in the Bourn Hall contract provide that the embryos are held for two years only, after which time the clinic renegotiates with its "parents" further retention. Any stored embryo will be reimplanted *only* in its mother, who must be married or in a stable heterosexual relationship at the time of the reimplantation. The replacement must be within "the competence of the scientific or medical staff."[45] A final clause deals with the use of embryos not needed for the purpose of reimplantation. With the consent of the parents involved, these may be used at Bourn Hall for research purposes. This has become one of the most contentious of the immediate issues thrown up by the various work in this field. The link between embryo research and IVF and embryo transfer is inseparable, they are the "core techniques of the biotechnical goldmine,"[46] and the wider question of research needs briefly to be addressed here.

One infertility treatment researcher has suggested that there are presently five important reasons for the promotion of research on embryos. These he gives as,

(i) the improvement of existing infertility treatments for both male and female patients,

(ii) the investigation of infertility when the causes are not apparent,

(iii) the deepening of understanding about miscarriages, whether through recurrent abortions or placental insufficiency; of the 100,000 women who suffer miscarriage each year in the UK little is known of the causes,

(iv) the improvement of techniques of contraception; early foetal development expresses proteins which are seen as one of the most promising avenues to fertility control vaccines.[47] The introduction of new forms of chemical and hormonal contraceptives is said to depend on embryo research to assess their potential impact on foetuses conceived by those using the new techniques,

(v) the reduction of genetic disease; about 14,000 babies die each year as a result of genetic disease and a much larger number are born with genetic handicaps.[48]

Other commentators have been more explicit in their aspirations, suggesting that the uses to which embryo research might contribute include not only fertility research, but also the alleviation of haemophilia, sickle cell anaemia, cystic fibrosis, the treatment of people whose bone marrow had been destroyed through radiation therapy following nuclear accident, and other forms of tissue grafting, where donated foetal tissue might be used to replace damaged brain, liver and pancreatic tissue. What is clear is that the use of embryo research in infertility is only "the first practical application of embryo research."[49] Developments in molecular cell biology are adding dimensions which ethicists and lawyers have yet hardly to address; for example embryo biopsy, where one or two cells from the pre-embryo are examined before implantation using DNA probes to investigate for the presence of a particular genetic disease.[50] Professor of Genetics, Derek Roberts, has reported that embryo research carries new possibilities for eliminating genetic disorders, such as chromosome surgery for Down's Syndrome, embryo donation for Turner's syndrome and gene replacement for Huntingdon's chorea and retinoblastoma.[51] The first cloning of human genes in 1977[52] has been followed by a vast increase in knowledge of common inherited disease and two major practical applications; attempts to improve the prevention and treatment of single gene defects (such as Huntingdon's and Alzheimer's diseases and phenylketonuria) and new approaches to polygenic conditions such as coronary heart disease. Similarly with inherited biochemical disease, such as haemophilia or muscular dystrophy, or chromosomal abnormalities such as Down's Syndrome, many of the relevant techniques are already in use for diagnostic purposes, and their adaptation and implementation as treatment is nearing.[53]

Several attempts have already been made in the British Parliament to prohibit or limit any research which involves the human embryo. In various guises, the Unborn Children (Protection) Bill—first brought to the House of Commons by Enoch Powell in February 1985[54] would seek to criminalise the creation, storage or use of a human embryo for any purpose other than to enable a child to be carried by a specified woman. In each case, a registered medical practitioner would have to apply in writing for the consent of the Secretary of State to the fertilisation of human ovum *in vitro*, and that authority would only be forthcoming if the Secretary was satisfied as to the arrangements made for the procedure and the competence and desirability of the medical personnel to be involved. Failure to observe these provisions would expose those who had procured the fertilisation to unlimited fines and up to two years imprisonment for conviction on indictment, or to a maximum six months imprisonment and fines not in excess of the statutory maximum for summary conviction.

The immediate impetus for the initial Bill was then MP Enoch Powell's reading of the Warnock Report. There, it had been proposed that licensed research should be permissible on human embryos for up to 14 days beyond fertilisation.[55] Edwards has reported that he never retains embryos for more than nine days and the Voluntary Licensing Authority remarked in their first Report that they understood that it has not been possible to keep human embryos alive for more than nine or ten days beyond fertilisation.[56] The Bills as drafted have been limited in what they would achieve, if their real force is aimed at the prevention of research. It is already possible to "harvest" fertilised eggs up to 20 days later from within the uterus; the cells in the petri dish may not survive (what has been dubbed loosely "abortion *in vitro*") and may then yield research potential in the same way that foetal tissue does now following abortion.[57] There are indeed, some embryos which it might be thought unethical to implant. For example, Williamson has suggested that "where ova are fertilised *in vitro*, it often happens that two sperm enter a single egg, giving a triploid embryo. Such an embryo is non-viable, and no one would reimplant it."[58] In these cases, the embryonic material if it is non-viable, could be made available for research purposes, and allow the dilemma posed by research on otherwise viable embryos to be sidestepped.

More contentious is the difficulty experienced by some researchers with the Warnock Committee's proposal that research on embryonic material should be permitted, but only until the 14th day after fertilisation has been completed. Organo-genesis occurs for the most part between 14 and 28 days of embryonic development; "it is the area of research, which is central to the understanding of congenital malformation, which-...would be most inhibited were a strict 14 day rule to be implemented."[59] The Government White Paper,[60] published in November 1987 in response to the Department of Health & Social Security's Consultative Document[61] issued following the Warnock Committee's Report, displays an astonishing vacill-ation on this point. Or perhaps it is more accurately characterised as a recognition that, politically, there are few votes to be gained in the cause of embryo research, wherever it is directed, but powerful social and moral communities to be antagonised and alienated along with their accompanying votes, if the "sanctity of life" doctrine in its most full expression becomes amenable to algebraic declension.

The White Paper announces that in the area of embryo research alone, alternative draft clauses are to be presented to Parliament for legislative consideration. One draft clause, aimed at prohibiting research with or on the human embryo, will constitute it a criminal offence to "carry out any procedures...other than those aimed at preparing the embryo for transfer to the uterus of a woman; or those carried out to ascertain the suitability of that embryo for the intended transfer." The clause which facilitates such broader research provides that a further exception to any criminal provisions will be permitted where the research is carried out "as part of a project specifically licensed by the SLA."[62] The

Statutory Licensing Authority is the proposed regulatory body which would oversee all developments and practices in the field of human fertilisation and embryology. It closely parallels the model suggested by the Warnock recommendations and anticipated by the Voluntary Licensing Authority established by two of the professional interest groups in the area, the Medical Research Council and the Royal College of Obstetricians and Gynaecologists in 1985. In neither case, however, would it be an offence to freeze embryos with the intention of their later transfer, nor to allow the embryos to perish if they were not to be transferred where, for example, an abnormality had been detected.

The White Paper nowhere provides, as the Unborn Children (Protection) Bills have done, that the embryos should be transferred only to a named woman. These earlier proposals would have entailed a separate application by a practitioner licensed specifically by the Secretary of State each time the transfer of an embryo was proposed, with any such permission given for a limited period of four months on each application.

Whichever of the avenues identified by the White Paper is followed, the signposts on the limitations on any permitted research are clearer. If any research is to be permitted, it will be for a period of 14 completed days from the time when the egg and the sperm are placed together for fertilisation. In computing this period, any time during which the embryo or pre-embryo spends in storage will be discounted.[63] The 14 day period, that favoured by the Warnock Committee, relates to specific understanding about human embryogenesis. It is at this stage that what is known as the "primitive streak" forms. This is the first of several identifiable features which form in and from the embryonic disc; the time when previously uncommitted embryonic cells in the epiblast layer of the embryonic plate pile up to make a groove "through which they move to give rise to a third layer of cells in the interior of the embryonic plate."[64] Most frequently, a single primitive streak will develop, marking the position of one embryo; occasionally two primitive streaks develop, evidencing the last stage at which monozygotic twins with shared amnion and placenta can result, and sometimes no streak appears because, for example, the embryonic plate contains too few cells, and no embryo results and the pregnancy ends.

If Parliament decides that any such licensed research is to be permitted, the White Paper proposes strict ethical and temporal limits on its conduct. Any SLA licence would be for a maximum period of two years, the research would have to be for a clearly

defined and stated aim, and the written consent of the gamete or
embryo donors obtained. As a condition of grant, the SLA would
have to be satisfied that the project aimed to bring about advances
in diagnostic or therapeutic techniques or fertility control, was
scientifically valid and that "adequate consideration to the
feasibility of achieving the aims of the project without the use of
human embryos" had been demonstrated.[65] The proposed legislation will also designate areas of prohibited research, which may be
reviewed parliamentarily from time to time. A further condition of
any licence would be an undertaking that work did not trespass
into these areas, which include cloning, the transfer of human
embryos to the uterus of another species or vice versa, and
embryonic gene structure modification, aimed at producing
artificially human beings with predefined characteristics, an
advanced form of eugenesis. One form of trans species fertilisation
will be permitted under very limited and strictly regulated
circumstances; that is where human sperm is used to penetrate the
egg of another species (commonly a hamster) in order diagnosti-
cally to assess the potency of the human male sperm. This, and
only this may be countenanced by the SLA "only in connection
with the assessment or diagnosis of sub-fertility before the
completion of the fertilisation process."[66]

The conundrum which recent work in human embryology and
the proposals which the White Paper now advances is neatly
exposed by Jonathan Glover;

> "If we can make positive changes at the environmental level,
> and negative changes at the genetic level (breeding out our
> 'faults' or 'anomalies') why should we not make positive
> changes at the genetic level?"[67]

One response has been suggested by Renate Duelli Klein, who has
pointed up some perceived hazards and possibilities of such
continued research. She has argued that new reproductive
technologies, epitomised by IVF and embryo transfer, are
undesirable and irresponsible because they are based on the idea
of a "technological fix" for a complex matrix of socio-economic,
iatrogenic and psychological problems; the need to have a
biological child of one's own, the production of children to order:

> "The new reproductive technologies are never exposed as
> technopatriarchy's obsession with conquering what is possibly
> the last great frontier—controlling the production of the
> human species (and finally all human life on earth)—by means

of... making us as alienated from our children as men have always been."[68]

This last observation is a purposeful recall of the arguments of Mary O'Brien who, in *The Politics of Reproduction*,[69] distinguishes the "reproductive consciousness" of women and men. For the man, she describes genetic continuity as largely an idea; reproduction beginning with the alienation of the male's sperm from his body and only nine months later there being any reassimilation into the reproductive process. For the woman, reproductive consciousness is delineated as a genetic continuity through the growth of the child within her and her active labouring process of giving birth. She argues that present developments, (and embryo transfer combined with some form of surrogate pregnancy, in particular), hold the potential radically to alter the reproductive experience of women, progressively providing for them the kind of discontinuity experienced by men. The struggle over various high technology interventions in birth—the presenting issue in the Wendy Savage affair—illustrates that some women value the reproductive consciousness that childbirth gives. IVF, especially if accompanied by routine caesarian section, reduces that experience, and embryo transfer may do so further.

The use of techniques such as IVF and embryo and egg freezing is far from a routinized practice in 1988. However, once the techniques are perfected they can be conducted with much greater distance from a woman's body. In other words, the fear is that

" ... a live woman won't be necessary at all as long as her eggs have been frozen which can then be stored in the lab and thawed, matured and fertilised at a convenient time."[70]

The force of this particular strand of apocalyptic feminist analysis is that it throws back into relief something which the embryo experiment argument has almost allowed to occlude; that embryos have limited physical potential without the prospect of reimplantation into a woman's womb.

What Edward Yoxen has identified as "an over individualised notion of the embryo," its genetic and developmental properties, has led to the virtual exclusion of concern with the embryo's necessary relatedness to another being:

" ... human embryos, even when they are fertilised *in vitro*, derive from ova which are formed within a woman's body and must be replaced within a woman's body to develop further.

Even embryos to be used in research are only available for research because a woman has made them available, hopefully with her informed consent. In this context, as also in *in vitro* fertilisation, her feelings are . . . more important than the moral status of the embryo cell system."[71]

Of course, as Yoxen recognises, this does not mean that the embryo (or pre-embryo as the pre-14 day conceptus is often now called),[72] has no moral status at all, nor no claim to moral recognition; it is a statement about priorities. The next sections seek to reconnoitre some of the signposts which have been suggested in this task of setting those priorities.

Technology and the Political Economy of Reproduction

The reproduction revolution brings in its wake many new and difficult choices. The categories of language and thought which we use are strained by the pace and propulsion of change. Technological "medicine" has been developed in such a way in the past thirty, twenty, ten, two years, that it is possible to envisage, and soon perhaps to create, concepts of birth, parenthood, and family faster than vocabulary can be brought to the aid of understanding. When, and how much, people are disturbed by things anomalous to their systems of classification is not, of course, susceptible to easy and cosy evaluation[73]; the "normal" and the "pathological" are cultural and historical specificities.[74] The response of the "Moral Right" to reproductive technologies emphasises the supposed security and certainty of traditional gender relations and family forms, cornerstones of the ideology of the New Right. These are held out as a place of safety from the technological stockmarket; with their promise of form, shelter, safety, rules and love—the taxonomy which Andrea Dworkin offers for the appeal of the known[75]—they trade upon the realisation that sexuality and reproduction touch deep chords of ambivalence, anxiety and fear in most of us.[76] And yet the role of these very relations and forms in maintaining domestic repression and inequality, in fracturing notions of equality, cooperation and reciprocity have themselves been well described and documented.[77]

Technology has, however, hastened our notion of self conception to the brink of an evolutionary surge. The notions of value and worth which we attach to individuals and social groups, the nature and meaning of fertility and the concept of the family are all implicated. The ensuing debate cuts into fundamental values, and increasingly the very institutions of maternity, paternity, mother-hood and fatherhood are subject to examination and re-evaluation.

The "plight" of the infertile is seen as legitimating the time, technology and resources expended on it; "one function of medicine is to alleviate the aberrations of nature. The treatment of infertility is intended to correct such an aberration and the natural situation is for a child to have two parents."[78] Leaving aside the apparent *non-sequitur*, there is the assumption that infertility is an exclusively biological *fact*, an aberration of nature, without a specific cultural backdrop or even an established aetiology.[79] I do not wish to deny the grief, anger, frustration, shame and waste which infertility generates.[80] It is worth recalling, however, that fertility is closely allied to the general position of women and men in society, and that infertility is as much a social *construct* as a biological fact;[81] in Barbara Schiterman's memorable phrase, "there is no pure biology in the socialised world."[82] But it is because women are defined by the medical and other professions almost exclusively as first and foremost *mothers* that the pursuit of infertility treatments has taken the shape and force which it has.[83] This is all part of, and indeed a continuation of the medicalisation and professionalisation of childbirth and child rearing,[84] which, when allied with control over the place of birth and the aggregation and allocation of resources represents a major transfer of power from women to men.[85] That, as Nikolas Rose has suggested, this is done in more subtle ways than through physical state coercion, should not obscure the realisation that the fear engendered by the usurpations is that "motherhood has become a male scientific achievement and is conducted according to male-devised rituals and regulations."[86] The effect of this has been to substitute for any other person medical technocrats as the arbiters and assessors of those "tragic choices" which all societies must presently make.

Guido Calabresi and Phillip Bobbitt have given us the vocabulary of the Tragic Choice: it is the intolerable choice demanded by conditions of scarcity between values accepted by a society as fundamental that mark some choices as tragic.[87] Childfulness and bodily integrity might be regarded as examples of two such values, although neither is uncontestable. According to Calabresi and Bobbitt, all tragic choices reveal two kinds of moving progression. These disclose, first, a society's oscillation between two sorts of decisions it must make regarding scarce goods; how much of the good there should be and who should have access to that good.[88] And, secondly, there exists the process of decision, rationalisation, and violence as quiet replaces anxiety to be replaced in turn by quiet, as a society evades, confronts and remakes the tragic choice:

> "Such a progression seeks to change our perception of the particular tragic dilemma. By making the result seem necessary, unavoidable, rather than chosen, it attempts to convert what is tragically chosen into what is merely a fatal misfortune."[89]

Reproductive technologies, seen through such a perspective exemplify clearly the nature of tragic choosing and demonstrate again that the politics of the family and the politics of the technological imperative interleave and interact. As the positions of women and men slowly change, the possibilities of separating sex from reproduction and nurturing form a *necessary* matrix for approaching and assessing reproductive technologies. Strategies which might follow from this, forms of second order rationalisation, include a de-emphasising and replacement of the privilege given to heterosexual relationships in official and personal discourse, a reworking of the dominant pictures of value, worth, fertility and infertility, and a new understanding of the quality of access to high and low level technologies. The extent to which these prescriptions may be seen to match positive analysis will help to indicate our position within the moving progressions. Two examples must here briefly serve to illustrate this point.

Technology and Motherhood

In 1970 Shulamith Firestone used the appreciation of the biological family unit as the consistent oppressor of women and children as the foundation stone for her argument that "for the first time in history, technology has created real preconditions for overthrowing these oppressive 'natural' conditions, along with their cultural reinforcements."[90] Yet, the overarching fear expressed more often since she wrote with all the reprotechnologies is that *under the control of men*, artificial reproduction is getting closer to being a distinctive capacity of the male: "future generations could be produced by men not reproduced by women."[91]

> "Despite their benefits for individual women, [reproductive technologies] also have the effect of carving out more and

more space/time for obstetrical "management" of pregnancy...they divert social resources from epidemiological
research into the causes of foetal damage. But the presumption of foetal "autonomy" ("patienthood" if not "personhood") is not an inevitable requirement of the technologies.
Rather, the technologies take on the meanings and uses they
do because of the cultural climate of foetal images and the
politics of hostility towards pregnant women and abortion."[92]

Firestone's analysis has, I think, been mediated in at least two
important ways since she wrote.

First, in the understanding of child*ful*ness as a choice with its
own internal validity as well as external affirmations. Allied to this
is the acknowledgment of the existence, if not their widespread
acceptance, of non-patriarchal forms of family life. There is, I
think, at least among those who have exercised an active, positive
choice to repudiate childfulness, women and men, a deeper
understanding and critical consciousness of the *production* of
childlessness as a cultural as well as biological function, and an
awareness and embracing of forms of nurturing which displace or
supersede the stable heterosexual family/childful unit.[93] When
Firestone was writing, the active assumption or repudiation of
childbearing was socially, culturally and sexually more limited
than today. There is no uncertain irony in the facets of recent state
policy, both in respect of the family and of employment practices,
which have threatened to recreate the world of enforced reproductive production as a means of negotiating enslaved and subsistence
means of existence.[94]

Secondly, Lesley Doyal,[95] Ann Oakley, Renate Duelli Klein and
many others have argued recently that the development of these
reproductive technologies present a *contradictory* choice for women.
Technically, some of the developments have increased the capacity
of women to control their own bodies; with some versions of cloning
and parthenogenesis the notion that reproduction belongs to women
would take on a new dynamic with the ability to reproduce without
the need of the patriarchal genetic. AID and even IVF have brought
the possibility of reproduction without most of the family structures
which for long were associated with it.[96] These "liberating" capacities and possibilities are, however, being offered at the potential
price of making those same bodies more available and accessible to
medical technocrats, giving greater power to that elite to exercise
control over women's lives. As Gena Corea writes, "[when] reproductive engineers have developed an artificial womb, they might
place the cultured embryo directly into the mother machine."[97]

And, while this conflict rages motherhood is glorified ideologically but attracts little esteem and support. It remains one of the lowliest and least rewarded jobs, calculated in 1986 to be worth £10,000 p.a. for 7 hours a day child care, with a consequent loss of earnings over 7 years to care and nurture two children of £54,000.[98] This report additionally estimates that a woman then returning to work loses a further £48,000 over her life through taking part rather than full-time work, and a further £32,000 lost because of the lower rates of pay for such work.

> "Our child-hating society turns mothering into a constant struggle with unsuitable, badly equipped buildings (shops, houses, public places), unfavourable work and training conditions, discriminatory educational opportunities, inadequate health care, and of course a host of related attitudes to mothers as "unreliable" workers because of their responsibility to take care of their children's needs."[99]

What Foucault has called the "hysterisation of women"[1] has social as well as medical aspects.

Reproductive Discrimination

As an illustration of the second order progression of the Tragic Choice, (who gets?) we may look again at two examples of what I earlier called "technological incest"; the basis on which the reproductive technologies are to be made available to those people who would seek to avail of them. Here, the Working Party of the Council for Science and Society observed, for example, that to include single women and lesbians in infertility treatment programmes "will increase social problems and child care and welfare" and be "a threat to normal family life."[2] Despite the unintentional irony attached to the threat to *social* life, not to the life of the individuals but to those who must deal with them, the negative assumptions here made are recalled by the Warnock Committee who opined that:

> "To judge from the evidence, many believe that the interests of the child dictate that it should be born into a home where there is a loving, stable, heterosexual relationship and that, therefore, the *deliberate* creation of a child for a woman who is not a partner in such a relationship is morally wrong...we believe that as a general rule it is better for children to be born into a two-parent family, with both father and mother,

although we recognise that it is impossible to predict with any certainty how lasting such a relationship will be."[3]

In other words, the Committee felt more comfortable with the idea of a child born into a home where the uncertainty of its parents' commitment to one another was mediated by the different genders of those whom it *assumed* would be that childs' primary carers, rather than to reason through the essential difficulties which it thought attached to child rearing in a family home where from birth the child lived in a homosexual or single carer environment. These negative assumptions cannot be borne out.

Susan Golombok, Ann Spencer and Michael Rutter,[4] have argued that the expectation that a mother's lesbianism would in itself increase the likelihood of psychiatric disorder arose largely from the assumption that the children living in lesbian households would be teased, ostracised or disapproved of by their peers, and that they would be adversely affected by this. In fact, no such differences could be detected when comparing the children of women who were now lesbian compared with those living in a single parent household; if anything, the tendency towards more behavioural and emotional problems lay the other way. The caveat in that important study, which also surveys some of the earlier literature, that "the findings cannot be applied to exclusively and permanently homosexual women who have become pregnant by means of AID,"[5] has to be balanced with their conclusion:

> "It remains very possible that there are effects on development (although they have not been empirically shown) of being brought up in a home that lacks any contact with men, in which there is a negative attitude towards things masculine, and in which there is active proselytizing of a homosexual way of life. While such a description may apply to a few lesbian households, it did not apply to those in our sample. We should cease regarding lesbian households as all the same. Like heterosexual households they differ greatly.... Perhaps it is the quality of family relationships and the pattern of upbringing that matters for psychosexual development, and not the sexual orientation of the mother."[6]

In a later essay, Susan Golombok, with John Rust[7] returns to argue that while it is clear that children in "fatherless families" are more likely to have emotional and behavioural problems, this is not, as often assumed, because of the absence of a father, but as a direct consequence of the poverty and isolation that these families have to endure.[8]

Golombok and Rust write:

> "Implicit in the view that children need fathers is the notion that the two-parent heterosexual family is the norm, and that any deviation from this ideal family structure is bound to cause problems for the child. But how normal is it? Around one in eight families with children in Britain are one-parent families. The large majority of these are headed by women and a growing percentage are unmarried. Is it really sensible to suppose that one and a half million or so children who are growing up in Britain today without fathers will be damaged by this experience? . . . it seems unlikely that the social and emotional development of AID and IVF children in fatherless families would be different from children who find themselves in heterosexual one-parent families or in lesbian families after they reach the age of two or three years."[9]

They suggest that the issue of lesbian access to AID and IVF is often phrased as a question of a child or children growing up in an environment with no males, in which there is no model of heterosexual relationships, negative attitudes to men, and pressures on the children to adopt atypical sex roles. And yet, as far as gender identity is concerned, there is no reason to suppose that lesbian women would bring up their sons as girls or their daughters as boys. There is, they caution, no empirical support for either psychoanalytic theories which posit that both boys and girls would develop atypically because of the lack of clearly differentiated father and mother roles; nor for some social learning theorists who have suggested that lesbian mothers might use a different pattern of reinforcement for male behaviour in boys, and that girls might be influenced by an atypical role model and might experience different patterns of reinforcement for sex-typed behaviours. As they conclude with what we may now regard as awful prescience:

> "Given the extent to which children are abused within the traditional system, surely the double standards which have so far permeated the debate about eligibility for AID and IVF should be recognised? . . . on the basis of 200 words which amount to dogma rather than argument, some women are to be denied the right to have children."[10]

End Notes

These two different types of argument, of the conflicting nature of technology for motherhood and of reproductive discrimination, parallel the oscillation which Tragic Choices force upon us. In attempting to come to terms with the values which reproductive technologies necessarily compromise, it seems to me that it is necessary to establish two clear priorities. First, power over the access to and quality of that technology must lie, collectively and individually, in the control of those faced with the consequences of the "success" or "failure" of these technologies. One move forward, whether with low or high technology, whether with "old" or "new," might be to convert the fear expressed by Women in Medicine in their submission to the Warnock Committee that "those who control the development of this technology are the ones who will benefit from it"[11], into an aspiration.

The past history of the development of medical technologies reveals their capacity for sexist, classist and racist uses, harboured within countervailing "benefits" saccharin-packed by the industrial interests which trade on scientific imperativism and imperialism.[12] In other words, if societal expectation, enshrined and encouraged by State policies, is that women continue to work in and within the family, then it is to them that control over the deployment and development of reproductive technologies belongs. If there is an officially sanctioned and practically realised reordering of public and private economies, then a more attenuated form of joint control might be appropriate. This I suggest is an urgent and necessary point of departure if we want to assimilate within the sexual identity located by Jeffrey Weeks[13] that notion of sexual intelligence identified and illustrated by Andrea Dworkin[14] as a counterweight to and complement of the more familiarly constructed concepts of creative and moral intelligencies.

The second imperative confronts directly the crucial question of reproductive "freedom" or "rights," which remains as the background for much of the debate. The limitations of rights arguments have been exhaustively exposed elsewhere, and the setting of the poor against the lame, the deaf against the ethnic group, the blind against the animal does not need presently to be rehearsed. As Whitbeck reflects, a rights based view of ethics see persons as social and moral atoms, actually or potentially in competition with one another; "if any attention is given to human relationships, it is assumed that they exist on a contractual or quasi contractual basis and that the moral requirements arising from them are limited to rights and obligations."[15] Perhaps it is here that the caution entered by Lucy Bland over the non-interchangeability of familiar terms again needs emphasis; maybe the rights which reproduction appeals to are not those of the public, political arena, but some different conception, based on a restructured notion of private, political autonomy.

The issue of reproductive choice has been less fully articulated. It has been the forcing ground on which many of the still limited successes for a more congenial picture of sexuality have been taken. But, even inherent within the argument from choice there appears to lie concealed a danger. As Robyn Rowland argues, it may be that the "right" to choose the sex of one's child, the "right" to use donor ova, the "right" to use a surrogate mother, and the "right" of the medical profession to service these rights,[16] have been used to ensure a lack of regulation other than by those who have the most vested interests in the continued exercise of other people's rights. The medical professionals whose status and budget is most closely tied to the continuing "success" and viability of "infertility" programmes, medical technology manufacturers, distributors, suppliers and servicers, all of whom depend for their continued financial health on the growth and nurturance of new and ever more sophisticated technology, are beholden to the continually reinforced desire of women to produce their "own" babies, and of men to have women produce "their" babies. Whereas, social and government intervention *is* what was called for and wanted in respect of abortion and sexuality, "is it what we want with reproductive technology. . . . What is the "right to choose" in this context?"[17] Here, the interconnectedness of the two priorities which I have identified is most clearly disclosed.

Whether the technologies which are under consideration are those now in the course of development, or those, such as pre-or post-conception sex selection or predetermination, which are technically well established, but of compromised ethical employment,[18] or whether they are more distant possibilities, such as ectogenesis or cloning, the stress or conflict, earlier identified by Moran,[19] is again evident. There is a direct interface between individual rights or autonomy and government policy, reflecting again the conflict of public and private domains, when these issues forced upon us by reprotechnologies fall to be, ever increasingly urgently, considered. Our evaluation of these reproductive alternatives, the tenets and moment of the "reproduction revolution" is not a neutral, non-gendered act, because this is not a "revolution" in the sense of something inspired and directed from below, but a diverse series of "medical advances" which insinuate and suffuse their values more indirectly. "The politics of reproductive technologies are constructed contextually, out of who uses them, how and for what purposes."[20] The nature of these "advances", is such that they can be pressed to augment the "panoptic technology" identified by Foucault,[21] through which nation states are concerned overtly and covertly, directly and indirectly, with the minutest details of the lives and deaths of their subjects.

Recall that Foucault identified in Bentham's plan for the Panoptican an architecture in which the subject is individualised and pathologised, such that

> "he is seen, but does not see; he is the object of information, never a subject in communication.... The Panoptican was also a laboratory, it could be used as a machine to carry out experiments, to alter behaviour, to train or correct individuals... It functions as a kind of laboratory of power..."[22]

As the nature and extent of personal birth, conception and sustenance becomes a global concern, the tragic choices of reproductive technology become, in fact, ways in which windows or curtains can be framed or drawn around our procreative and affective lives. Having the ability to take charge of the personal moments of one's own reproductive choices becomes an imperative way of thinking about and defining ourselves, or of enslaving ourselves and others. Before assessing reproductive technologies, it is necessary to have access to the knowledge and resources to judge its uses and their wisdom. It may be that that is precisely what the Tragic Choice will deny us.

Notes

This paper was given as a lecture at Middlesex Polytechnic in 1986, and I benefited from comments there; the discussion which followed its delivery as a Current Legal Problems seminar forced me to think more critically about some of the points I was making, and exposed deficiencies which it then had. Edward Yoxen of the Department of Science & Technology Policy, University of Manchester commented on an earlier draft and gave me some important lines of enquiry to pursue; my colleague Celia Wells has read various versions and attempted to ensure that I have clarified my ideas and their expression. I owe a particular debt to Frances Price of the Child Care & Development Group, University of Cambridge, and Jennifer Gunning of the Medical Research Council, who carefully read and corrected this essay and provided me with access to some of the more important recent medical literature. The usual caveats apply.

End Notes   49

[1] Antoine de Saint Exupéry, *Wind, Sand and Stars* (1939, 1975 ed.), pp. 39–40.
[2] Miriam David, "Moral and Maternal: the Family in the Right" in Ruth Levitas, (ed.), *The Ideology of the New Right*, (1986).
[3] Liz Kingdom, (1986) 1 *Disability, Handicap & Society* 113, at p. 116.
[4] Malcolm Wicks, "Enter Right; The Family Patrol Group," *New Society*, February 24, 1983.
[5] Jane Lewis, "The Politics of Motherhood in the 1980s: Warnock, Gillick and Feminists," (1986) 13 J. Law & Soc., 321 at p. 322–25.
[6] Lucy Bland, *Marxism Today*, September 1985, p. 21.
[7] Les Moran, "A Reading in Sexual Politics and Law," (1986) 8 *Liverpool Law Review* 83 at p. 84.
[8] Edward Yoxen, "Human Embryo Research: A Cause for Concern?", paper presented at the British Sociological Association conference, Leeds, April 1987, p. 4.
[9] Commenting on an earlier presentation of part of this present paper, Middlesex Polytechnic, March 1986.
[10] Nikolas Rose, "Beyond the Public/Private Division: Law, Power and the Family" in Peter Fitzpatrick and Alan Hunt, (eds.), *Critical Legal Studies*, (1987) 61 at 68.
[11] *Ibid.* p. 66.
[12] Lorraine Harding, "The Debate on Surrogate Motherhood: the Current Situation, Some Arguments and Issues: Questions Facing Law and Policy", (1987) J. Social Welfare Law, 37.
[13] D.H.S.S. *Review of Child Care Law*, (1985), §§ 15.12–25. § 15.25 contains the proposal that, in making a care order, the court must be satisfied that

> "there is likely to be a substantial deficit in the standard of health, development, or well-being which can reasonably be expected . . . and that the deficit or likely deficit is the result of the child not receiving or being unlikely to receive the care that a reasonable parent can be expected to provide . . . "(my emphasis).

[14] *Gillick* v. *West Norfolk and Wisbech A.H.A.* [1986] A.C. 112.
[15] *Supra*, note 7, pp. 89–90.
[16] (1983), p. 7.
[17] (1984).
[18] Cmnd. 9314, (1984).
[19] Jane Lewis, *supra*, note 5. The *Second Report of the Voluntary Licensing Authority for Human In Vitro Fertilisation and Embryology*, April 1987, Guideline 13(j), at p. 35, recommends that egg donors should be anonymous because "there are relationships with which the practice would be inadvisable." On this, see Frances Price, "Reproductive Technology" in Robert Lee and Derek Morgan, (eds.), *Birthrights: Law & Ethics at the Beginning of Life*, (1988, forthcoming).
[20] Edward Yoxen, *Unnatural Selection*, (1986), pp. 4–6.
[21] *Ibid.* p. 5.
[22] *Subject Women*, (1985 ed.), pp. 198–90.
[23] Ann Oakley, *Captured Womb*, (1985), p. 283.
[24] *Ibid.* p. 256.
[25] *Ibid.* p. 254.
[26] Michelle Stanworth, *Reproductive Technologies; Gender, Motherhood and Medicine*, (1987), p. 3.
[27] *Supra*, note 10, p. 67.
[28] Aldous Huxley, "Foreword," *Brave New World*, (1950 ed.), p. 8.

50   Technology and the Political Economy of Reproduction

29 This taxonomy is suggested by Renate Duelli Klein in her essay "What's 'new' about the 'new' reproductive technologies?" in G. Corea, *et. al.*, (eds.), *Man Made Women*; *How the New Reproductive Technologies affect Women*, (1985), 64, pp. 64–5.

30 *Ibid.* p. 67.

31 *Supra*, note 26, p. 4. The categorisation of reproductive technologies in this way can, of course, be challenged. Techniques for sex determination pre and post conception are well established and generally reliable; it is the ethical implications of some of the uses to which they are put that is problematic, see note 117, below. On the other hand, the 8.5 per cent. live birth rate for all IVF centres in the United Kingdom given by the VLA in its *Second Report, supra*, note 19, challenges the notion of "success" used here.

32 *Supra*, note 20, Chap. 2.

33 Robert Winston, *Infertility; A Sympathetic Approach*, (1986), p. 160. And see, (1986) 26 *Medicine, Science & Law* 82. There is a review by Seppela of *in vitro* fertilisation programmes in "The World Collaborative Report of In Vitro Fertilisation and Embryo Replacement: Current State of the Art in 1984", in M. Seppala and R.G. Edwards, (eds.), *In Vitro Fertilisation and Embryo Transfer*, (1985) 442 *Annals of the New York Academy of Science*, pp. 558–63. For more up-to-date analysis see (1988)(1) Fertility & Sterility, and *Third Annual Report of the Voluntary Licensing Authority for Human In Vitro Fertilisation and Embryology*, May 1988.

34 *Ibid.* p. 154.

35 Oral presentation, Newcastle University Philosophical Society Symposium, "Wider Implications of Research on Human Embryos", March 1986.

36 17.7 per cent. of women implanted via IVF have a successful term pregnancy following their treatment in the Bourn Hall Clinic. American workers in the field are reputed to have described this ratio as the "take home baby rate;" Edwards, *supra*, note 35.

37 *Ibid. cf.* Winston, *supra*, note 34, p. 155.

38 Winston, *supra*, note 34, p. 106. This "check" is a visual one only, and surveys the aesthetic quality of the embryo, trying to identify peripheral structural deficiencies.

39 *First Report of the Voluntary Licensing Authority for Human In Vitro Fertilisation and Embryology*, April 1986, § 5.2.

40 *Ibid.* § 5.3.

41 *Supra*, note 35.

42 Progress, *Pamphlet on Embryo Research*, 1986.

43 *The Guardian*, October 4, 1987, p. 3 carried a report of a recovery of 47 eggs, but this is presently most unusual.

44 *VLA Second Report supra*, note 19, in guideline 12, at p. 35, provides that "(a) if the IVF procedure is used no more than three pre-embryos should be transferred in any one cycle, unless there are exceptional clinical reasons when up to four pre-embryos may be replaced per cycle, (b) if the GIFT procedure is used no more than three or exceptionally four eggs should be introduced to the fallopian tubes." For refusing to abide by this guideline, Professor Ian Craft's programme at the Humana Hospital, London has had its VLA licence withdrawn. John Keown has questioned the legality of some of these procedures, see (1987) 137 New L.J., pp. 1165–66. In Germany up to twelve pre-embryos have been transferred, and subsequently reduced to three foetuses, see Frances Price, *supra*, note 19, nn. 38–39.

45 Edwards has indicated that Bourn Hall would use this clause to avoid any "post-mortem" reimplantation of women following the death of their male partner.

This issue has surfaced in England, Australia and France, where in the latter, Corinne Parpalaix successfully petitioned the French courts for the return of her husband's sperm deposited in a sperm bank shortly before his death a few months earlier from cancer. She successfully argued that the deposited sperm implied a contract which did not breach her dead husband's right to physical integrity, as the State Prosecutor had contended. (August 1984) The sperm was duly returned to her. She failed to become pregnant. In the United Kingdom, the Infertility Services Ethical Committee of a northern District Health Authority refused to allow a widow to be artificially inseminated with the deep frozen sperm of her deceased husband. The husband had been warned before his death that the cancer treatment he was about to undergo might leave him infertile and had in consequence left a written and video taped request that his widow be inseminated following his death. The Ethics Committee took the view that the man had had no legal dominion over his genetic material and that his widow had no legal right to receive it. Living human tissue, said the Committee, cannot belong to anybody; see the discussion of this case by Liz Kingdom, "Birthrights: Equal or Special" in Lee and Morgan, *supra*, note 19. Clearly, there are very important legal and ethical issues involved here, and they present a fine contrast with reports of instances where brain stem dead women have been artificially maintained on "life" support machines until it is thought opportune to deliver the foetus, which they were carrying on death, by Ceasarian section. I attempt to deal with these problems in a separate paper, "Posthumous Children: The Law and Ethics of Life After Death."

46 Renate Duelli Klein, "IVF: For Whose Benefit?—At Whose Expense?", paper presented at the European Critical Legal Studies Conference, London, April 1986, p. 12.

47 This point is made by Bob Williamson, "Research Needs and the Reduction of Severe Congenital Disease" in *Human Embryo Research: Yes or No?*, (1986), 105, at p. 110.

48 *Supra*, note. 34, pp. 167–68.

49 Edwards, *supra*, note 35. Foetal tissue is obtained from abortus material and has already been used experimentally for the relief of Parkinson's Disease and immune deficiency in infants. Gene therapy of the sort discussed in the text would be prohibited by the proposed legislation outlined in the White Paper, *Human Fertilisation and Embryology: A Framework for Legislation*, Cm. 259, (1987), § 28–42. If perfected, however, therapy of the sort envisaged could only be applied to the very early embryo while its cells were still totipotential.

50 *Supra*, note 47, Wetherall *et. al.*, pp. 116–18, Braude, p. 116, McLaren, p. 117.

51 Presentation to the Newcastle Philosophical Society Symposium, *supra*, note 35.

52 *Supra*, note 47, p. 105.

53 *Supra*, note 51.

54 And by others in 1986 and 1987.

55 *Supra*, note 18, § 11.22. The choice of 14 days was not arbitrary. This relates to what is now known of the early stages of development of the fertilised egg. It is suggested that up until 14 days it is not possible to know whether the fertilisation has produced anything which will develop beyond a cluster of cells. This cluster has become known as the conceptus, zygote or pre-embryo. About six days after fertilisation, this cluster of cells begins to attach itself to the uterine wall. A group of small cells at the centre of the cluster then begins to organise itself into a flat, oval two-tiered shape—the embryonic plate. Around the 14th day following fertilisation, if the cells have met no other unfavourable conditions in the uterus there takes place what is regarded as the crucial transformation, the development in the embryonic plate of a groove into which a third layer of cells migrates. This

groove is called the "primitive streak." For an overview of the scientific literature, see *Warnock Report*, §§ 11.2–7 and Penelope Leach, "Human *In Vitro* Fertilisation*," Annex 3, Voluntary Licensing Authority Report, *supra*, note 39, p. 39, 39–40, and text accompanying note 64, below. It is the development of the streak which is being increasingly fixed upon as the time when the rubicon is crossed between molecular matter and a potential human being.

[56] *Supra*, note 39.

[57] See "The Use of Foetuses and Foetal Material for Research" and the accompanying Code of Practice, H.M.S.O., 1972 (the Peel Report) and *Warnock*, § 11.18, note. 2.

[58] *Supra*, note 47, p. 110.

[59] *Ibid.* p. 109.

[60] *Human Fertilisation and Embryology*, *supra*, note 49.

[61] *Legislation on Human Infertility Services and Embryo Research: A Consultation Paper*, Cm. 46, (1986).

[62] *Supra*, note 49, § 30.

[63] *Ibid.* §§ 31–34.

[64] *Supra*, note 47, McLaren, at pp. 9–11.

[65] *Supra*, note 49, § 35.

[66] *Ibid.* § 42, deemed to be the two cell stage.

[67] *What Sort of People Should There Be?*, 1984, p. 46.

[68] Klein, *supra*, note 46, p. 3.

[69] (1981).

[70] *Klein, supra*, note 46, p. 5. And see Klein, *supra*, note 29, pp. 66–70.

[71] *Supra*, note 8, p. 29, and see Barbara Katz Rothman, *The Tentative Pregnancy*, (1986), p. 114, cited in Rosalind Pollack Petchesky, "Foetal Images: the Power of Visual Culture in the Politics of Reproduction," in Stanworth, *supra*, note 26, p. 57, at p. 63.

[72] *Supra*, note 47, McLaren, pp. 8–10.

[73] *Supra*, note 67, p. 40.

[74] Georges Canguilhem, *The Normal and the Pathological*, (1949, 1978 ed.).

[75] Andrea Dworkin, *Right Wing Women: The Politics of Domesticated Females*, (1982).

[76] Lucy Bland, *supra*, note 6, p. 21.

[77] See, for example, Jocelyn A. Scutt, (ed.), *Violence in the Family*, (1980).

[78] *Supra*, note 16, p. 7.

[79] Lesley Doyal with Immogen Pennell, *The Political Economy of Health*, (1981), p. 229.

[80] Naomi Pfeffer and Anne Wollett, *The Experience of Infertility*, (1983); Miriam Mazor and Harriet Simons, (eds.), *Infertility: Medical, Emotional and Social Considerations*, (1984).

[81] Doyal and Pennell, *supra*, note 79 and Germaine Greer, *Sex and Destiny*, (1984), p. 56 *et seq.*

[82] Barbara Sichtermann, *Femininity; the Politics of the Personal*, (1983, 1986 ed.), p. 63.

[83] R. Albury, "Who Owns the Embryo?" in Rita Arditti, Renate Duelli Klein and Shelley Minden, (eds.), *Test-Tube Women*, (1984), p. 54, at pp. 57, 65.

[84] Ann Oakley, "Women, Science and Reproduction; Some Terms in a Debate," paper given at the BAAS Conference, Bristol, September 1986, p. 3.

[85] Wendy Savage, Oral Presentation to the British Association for the Advancement of Science, Bristol, September, 1986.

[86] *Reproductive Wrongs*, (1984), p. 6.

[87] *Tragic Choices*, (1978), pp. 17–18.

[88] This, of course, requires decisions to be made as to how these second order

decorations are to be made.

[89] *Supra*, note 87, p. 22.

[90] *The Dialectic of Sex*, (1970), p. 183.

[91] Dale Spender, *For the Record; The Making and Meaning of Feminist Knowledge*, (1984), p. 93.

[92] Petchesky, *supra*, note 71, p. 64. For a recent example, see *In Re F. (In Utero.)*, (1988) discussed in Morgan "Judges on Delivery" (1988) J.S.W.L. 164.

[93] For a discussion of these possibilities see Noami Pfeffer, "Artificial Insemination, In Vitro Fertilisation and the Stigma of Infertility" in Michelle Stanworth, *supra*, note 26, p. 81, at pp. 82–83.

[94] See, for example, Beatrix Campbell, *Wigan Pier Revisited*, (1984).

[95] *Supra*, note 81.

[96] For example. *The Independent*, December 11, 1987. The BPAS estimates an increase from 5 to 11 per cent. of single women choosing to retain that status following childbirth. The legislation proposed in the White Paper, *supra*, note 49, § 27, would render it an offence to carry out insemination without a licence from the proposed Statutory Licensing Authority.

[97] "The Reproductive Brothel" in Corea, *supra*, note 29, p. 49.

[98] Jo Roll, *Babies and Money: Birth Trends*, 1986, Family Policy Studies Centre. Heather Joshi, "The Cash Opportunity Costs of Childbearing: An Approach to Estimation Using British Data," Discussion Paper series no. 208, Centre for Economic Policy Research, (1988), estimates that a typical loss of earnings attributable to child birth is twenty times the typical woman's salary as at age twenty four; "the typical mother who gives up work for several years to rear two children, forgoes £122,000 of income . . . ". This figure comprises, £54,000 loss of earnings over eight years; £48,000 loss due to part time rather than full time work; £10,000 loss in nine years work at lower pay; £5,000 attributable to low pay in the period when the "typical" woman works part time anyway.

[99] Klein, *supra*, note 29, p. 66.

[1] *The History of Sexuality*, (1984 ed.), p. 104.

[2] *Supra*, note 17.

[3] Warnock *supra*, note 18, § 2.11, and to similar effect, §§ 4.16 and 5.10.

[4] "Children in Lesbian and Single Parent Households: Psychosexual and Psychiatric Appraisal" (1983) 24(4) J. Child Psychol. Psychiat, 551.

[5] *Ibid.* p. 569.

[6] *Ibid.*

[7] "The Warnock Report and Single Women: What About the Children?" (1986) J. Medical Ethics, 182.

[8] On which see, for example, E. Ferri, *Growing Up in a One Parent Family*, (1976).

[9] *Supra*, note 7, p. 184.

[10] *Ibid*, p. 185.

[11] Cited in Jane Lewis, *supra*, note 5, p. 341 note 65.

[12] For example, Doyal and Pennell, *supra*, note 81 and Phillida Bunkle, "Calling the Shots? The International Politics of Depo-Provera" in Rita Arditta *et. al.*, *supra*, note. 83.

[13] *Sexuality and Its Discontents*, (1985), p. 185.

[14] *Supra*, note 75, pp. 180 *et seq.*

[15] "The Moral Implications of Regarding Women as People: New Perspectives on Pregnancy and Personhood," in W. Bondeson *et. al.*, (eds.), *Abortion and The Status of the Foetus*, (1983), pp. 249–50.

[16] Robyn Rowland, "Motherhood, alienation and the issue of 'choice' in sex preselection," in Corea, *et. al.*, *supra*, note 29.

[17] *Ibid.*

[18] For recent examples of the controversy to which these techniques give rise, see *The Independent*, January 4, 1988; *The Guardian*, January 4, 1988, discussed in Morgan "Foetal Sex Identification, Abortion and the Law; (1988) *Family Law* 108.

[19] Moran, *supra*, note 7.

[20] Petchesky, *supra*, note 71, p. 77.

[21] Michel Foucault, *Discipline and Punish*: *The Birth of the Prison*, (1977, trans., Alan Sheridan), pp. 195 *et. seq.*

[22] *Ibid.* pp. 200–202.

Sterilising the Mentally Handicapped

M.D.A. FREEMAN

The legal year has seen England's judges wading through a moral quagmire as novel ethical questions have been paraded before them: surrogacy issues,[1] the "rights" of a father to stop his girlfriend having an abortion,[2] the extent to which account should be taken of harm suffered by the child of a heroin addict before birth,[3] the freedom of an IVF clinic to deny treatment to an ex-prostitute[4] and, of course, the plight of Jeanette.[5] All these decisions received wide media coverage and were subjected to criticism, not all of it well-focussed and some of it ill-informed. The then Lord Chancellor, Lord Hailsham, was forthright in his condemnation of, what he considered to be, intemperate criticism.[6] I was one of the critics, the one, indeed, whose remark on the *Today* programme[7] that the Court of Appeal decision in the Jeanette case was "Nazi-like" (the proposition put to me was it was "Orwellian") reverberated round the globe. I do not consider this comment intemperate or unfounded, but it was a snap reaction at 7.20 (or thereabouts) and it was made without the benefit (if that is the right word) of the Court of Appeal judgments. I return to *Re B.* now with the wise words of the editor of the *Journal of Medical Ethics* in my mind. He wrote in a leading article that: "We must be even more than usually meticulous about subjecting our gut 'response' to the searchlight of critical moral reasoning."[8] There can be few better test-beds of the need to inject critical moral thinking into questions of law and medicine than the Jeanette saga.[9]

But, whatever the facts of *Re B.*, and Lord Bridge in the House of Lords was right to say that in many quarters there had been an "erroneous appreciation of the facts,"[10] it is necessary to put the sterilisation issue into its wider historical and cultural context. Only then can the sense of moral outrage which greeted the Jeanette decision be appreciated. The remark of La Forest J. in *Re Eve* (Canada's recent counterpart to *Re B.*) that "social history clouds our vision"[11] is all too true.

Sterilisation: the Historical Context

I will start with a quotation from a reform school administrator in the United States. "Many people" he said, "are 'put off' by what Hitler did in Germany; but, again, you have to be practical."[12] I find this remark utterly distasteful but it is essentially what the courts were saying in *Re B*. But sterilisation for eugenic or other social control purposes neither begins nor ends in Nazi Germany. As an ideology eugenics can be traced back to 1869 and, whisper it not too loudly, to the portals of that bastion of liberalism, University College London.[13] The first attempt to pass a law mandating involuntary sterilisation was made in Michigan in 1897.[14] It failed. But vasectomies were already being used at an Indiana state reformatory (they started in about 1890). A Dr Sharpe employed this procedure on 600 to 700 boys.[15]

In 1907 Indiana became the first American state to pass a compulsory sterilisation statute. Similar statutes were soon enacted in Washington, California and Connecticut and, by the time the eugenics movement reached its peak in the 1920's, 28 states in the USA had passed involuntary sterilisation laws. A number of them were declared unconstitutional: some were impugned as "cruel and unusual" punishment; others fell foul of "due process" or "equal protection under the law" clauses. But in 1927 the Supreme Court decided *Buck* v. *Bell*.[16]

Carrie Buck was, in the language of the day, "feeble-minded," the daughter of a mother alleged to be feeble-minded and the mother herself, research has shown, of a daughter of above average intelligence (though in the law report she is described as an "illegitimate feeble minded child"). Her proposed sterilisation under a Virginia statute was challenged on "due process" and "cruel and unusual" punishment grounds. The court's response was it was not done as a punishment, and that in fact sterilising her enabled her to be released to the community—an argument often still heard today, the reverberations of which also echo in *Re B*. Due process and equal protection arguments were also rejected. The sterilisation statute was upheld as constitutional. The only opinion was given by Justice Holmes. His judgment is not good news for the "bad woman."[17] He noted that the attack was "not upon the procedure but upon the substantive law." However, he argued:

"We have seen more than once that the public welfare may call upon the best citizens for their lives. It would be strange if

it could not call upon those who already sap the strength of
the State to make lesser sacrifices, often not felt to be such by
those concerned. In order to prevent our being swamped with
incompetents, it is better for all the world if instead of waiting
to execute degenerate offspring for crime or to let them starve
for their imbecility, society can prevent those who are
manifestly unfit from continuing their kind. The principle that
sustains compulsory vaccination is broad enough to cover
cutting the fallopian tubes. Three generations of imbeciles are
enough."[18]

Those familiar with Lord Denning's remarks in *Bravery* v.
Bravery[19] may wonder what it is about sterilisation that brings out
the worst in great judges.

Justice Holmes's opinion has been castigated so often that
anything I might say about it is otiose. A couple of points,
however, should be made if only to guide us through the thickets
of the Jeanette case. First, Holmes's analysis, in particular his
analogies, is weak (the temptation is to describe it as "sub-
standard" whatever the implications of this might be!). His
language is intemperate and value-laden. The war analogy is
fatuous: the enemy who kills our soldiers is in no way comparable
to the progeny of a mentally handicapped person who may require
state support. The principle behind compulsory vaccination (a
policy, incidentally, opposed by the very Social Darwinists who
advocated eugenics)[20] cannot encompass involuntary sterilisation,
any more than it would the cutting off of the hands of habitual
thieves: the quality of the intrusion is totally different. Secondly, it
needs to be said that Holmes was far too readily convinced that
due process had been observed. It surely behoves any judge
sanctioning the deprivation of a basic human right to invoke higher
standards of scrutiny than in the ordinary case.

There have been a number of significant cases in the USA since
Buck v. *Bell*.[21] There have been attempts to reverse the decision.
That this has not happened is in part attributable to the fact that
the line of argument has changed. Eugenics (or rather
"negative"[22] eugenics) is out of fashion: instead, the appeal is
grounded on the burden placed on society by the need to care for
the handicapped. The most interesting of the recent cases is *North
Carolina Association for Retarded Children* v. *State of North
Carolina* in 1976.[23] The statute challenged authorised both
voluntary and involuntary sterilisations. There was a duty to
institute sterilisation proceedings when the relevant official felt it
was either in (i) the best interests of the retarded person or (ii) the

public at large or (iii) where the retarded person would be likely, unless sterilised, to procreate children with a tendency to serious physical, mental or nervous disease or deficiency or would be unable to care for the child or (iv) when the next of kin or legal guardian of the retarded person "requests" that he file the petition.   The court found (iv) irrational and irreconcilable with (i), (ii) and (iii). But it thought the first three provisions made out "a complete and sensible scheme."[24] The fourth, however, granted to the retarded person's next of kin or legal guardian "the power of a tyrant."[25] The scheme was thus found constitutional with the exception of the fourth provision. The language and ideology of Holmes's "incantation" was rejected. "Medical and genetical experts," the Court noted, "are no longer sold on sterilization to benefit either retarded patients or the future of the Republic."[26] The case is also significant for containing a number of general propositions about the origins of mental retardation, about expression of sexuality, about the ability of the handicapped to use contraceptive methods. Finally, the opinion holds that in rare unusual cases it can be medically determined that involuntary sterilisation is in the best interests of either the mentally retarded persons, or the state, or both.

A lot of people have been sterilised in the USA pursuant upon the compulsory programmes depicted here. By 1964, by which time the programmes had long passed their peak, 63,678 such sterilisations had taken place.[27] Those sterilised were mainly young women and for the large part they were poor and came from socio-economically   and   culturally   deprived   environments. Whether it was, as Gonzales indicates,[28] a popular way of controlling reproduction, it certainly was a convenient method for controlling the reproductive urges of the populace. Given the population concerned and the imperfections of classification, the dangers of labelling with sterilisation merely an incident of stigmatisation were difficult to overcome. The evidence suggests they were not surmounted.[29]

In the light of all this, it is somewhat surprising that forced sterilisation policies should be associated with Nazi Germany. But the reputation is deserved for no political system has pursued the policy with greater vigour or ruthlessness.[30] The Nazi compulsory sterilisation law dates from 1933, the very outset of the Third Reich and long before the Nuremberg Laws. The 1933 law created "hereditary health courts" made up of a district judge and his physicians to supplement, what was called, the "Law on the Prevention of Hereditary Diseases in Future Generations." A variety of diagnoses could lead to forced sterilisations including hereditary blindness or deafness, epilepsy, Huntingdon's disease and alcoholism. Many others designated "anti-social," such as Gypsies or, what were called, "Rhineland bastards" (children conceived after the First World War by French North African occupation troups) were also sterilised. A gradual shift towards measures aimed at racial elimination is evident here, as it became all too evident later.[31] The USA and Nazi Germany are but two of the countries in which involuntary sterilisation policies have been pursued.[32] Most recently, under Indira Gandhi, Indian governments have used sterilisation as a method of population control; in theory persons agreed to be sterilised (some, I seem to remember, in return for gifts of transistor radios) but in practice there is no doubt that forced sterilisation was carried out on a wide scale.

In England there has been surprisingly little discussion of sterilisation. The "Sotos Syndrome" case in 1975 (*Re D.*)[33] commanded a lot of public attention and Heilbron J.'s decision was generally acclaimed. But the Sheffield girl in *Re D.* was not the first English victim, or even the first in Sheffield. The chance intervention by an educational psychologist and the financial support of the NCCL for once converted a private matter into a public concern. Just how many young persons have been sterilised in Britain is something that will never be known. Dr. David Owen in 1975 said the Ministry of Health kept no comprehensive statistics. He quoted figures from two out of 14 regional health authorities.[34] According to *The Sun* in September 1975 the DHSS believed that in 1973 and 1974 11 girls and four boys under 16 had been sterilised and 29 girls and 34 boys of between 16 and 18.[35] Figures in the *Journal of Medical Ethics* do not tally with these. It is indicated there (by Sir George Porter) that at least 14 sterilisations were performed in this period on under 16 years olds and another 22 on those in the age range 16 to 18.[36] According to the *Birmingham Evening Mail* (in January 1976) one West Midlands leading child psychiatrist had himself recommended twelve adolescents under 16 for sterilisation.[37] In *Re D.* there is reference to two sterilisations having been carried out in Sheffield.[38] Figures released by the Department of Health in March 1987 indicate that about 90 sterilisations are performed a year in England on females under 19. The Department is unable to break the figures down into those aged under 18, and those who have reached the age of majority, nor to give the reasons for the sterilisations.[39]

Re D. provoked "an outrage about human rights"[40] (how many had slipped through the protective net that saved *D*?). It also provoked the DHSS into formulating a Discussion Paper "Sterilisation of Children under 16 years of age" which, so far as I can tell, has now sunk without trace. It should have led to an agreed Code of Practice. It may be that interest in formulating such a code will have been re-activated by the *Jeanette* case. Without such a code, the only guidance will remain the legal decisions in *Re B.* and *Re D.*

The question of sterilisation has rarely claimed public attention. Was anyone really interested before the Sheffield case or between it and *Re B.*? It is very significant that Mason and McCall Smith, whose second edition of *Law and Medical Ethics* was published this year, devote barely two pages to the subject and, though they call sterilisation "a minefield of powerful objection,"[41] are able in 1987 to describe abortion as the law's only "major incursion into reproductive practices."[42] It is also, I think, worth observing that Lord Oliver in *Re B.* thought Jeanette's case raised "no general issue of public policy."[43]

I turn now to look at *Re B.*, and in doing so take backward glances to the "Sotos Syndrome" case, as well as envious looks across the Atlantic to Canada where the Supreme Court handed down last year a decision (*Re Eve*), which is in striking contrast to the Lords' ruling and reasoning.

Jeanette: How the Courts Reasoned

The facts of Jeanette's case are now well-known. Her chronological age was 17, her mental age five or six. She was exhibiting the normal sexual drive and inclinations for someone of her age. She is described as severely mentally handicapped and epileptic. It was said that she had no understanding of the connection between sex, pregnancy and birth; that she would not be able to cope with birth or care for a child. There was expert evidence that it was vital that she should not be permitted to become pregnant and that certain contraceptive drugs would react with drugs administered to control her mental instability and epilepsy. There was further evidence that it would be difficult, if not impossible, to place her on a course of oral contraceptive pills. The local authority, in whose care she was, applied for her to be made a ward of court and for leave for her to undergo a sterilisation operation. Her mother supported the application. So did Bush J. the Court of Appeal and the House of Lords. Why?

In reading the judgments (and speeches) there is a natural break between Bush J. and the Court of Appeal on the one hand and the House of Lords on the other. Though Dillon L.J. in the Court of

Appeal can describe it as an "anxious case,"[44] the public policy issues only emerge in the speeches of the Lords after the Court of Appeal's decision is subjected to critical attention in the media. But in terms of what is decided, there is essential continuity between all three courts. This was a wardship application and it is clear law that only one criterion should govern such applications: *viz*: that the minor's welfare is the first and paramount consideration.[45] It is, it has been said, "the golden thread" which runs through the wardship jurisdiction: welfare is considered "first, last and all the time."[46] All three courts rightly identified Jeanette's welfare as their only concern. This is most forcibly stated in the Lords, doubtless to counter criticism made of the earlier decisions, but it is clearly also Bush J.'s concern. "Welfare" assumes less profile in Dillon L.J.'s judgment (the only relatively full judgment in the Court of Appeal) but it clearly is at the root of his thoughts. The Lords use the expression "welfare," "best interests" and "benefit" interchangeably: although these are not identical conceptions, this is not something with which I will quibble. The Lords accordingly held that where it was for the welfare and in the best interests of the ward that she be sterilised, the Court had jurisdiction to authorise the operation. On the facts, they held it was. To Lord Hailsham the welfare of the ward in this case was the "only" consideration (there are, of course, cases where it is not,[47] but Lord Hailsham is not casting doubt on the exceptions). Similarly, for Lord Oliver the appeal was concerned "with one primary consideration and one alone, namely the welfare and best interest of this young woman."[48]

In *Re D.* Heilbron J.'s refusal to authorise the sterilisation of an 11 year old had been premised on its irreversible nature and the deprivation of "a basic human right," namely the right of a woman to reproduce.[49] None of the judges found any difficulty in distinguishing *Re D.* and, it is true, there are material differences. Lord Hailsham, indeed, contented himself in the belief that Heilbron J. would decide *Re B.* as he was now deciding it. As far as the "basic human right" is concerned, Bush J. expressed the reaction of all the judges: "one is in effect depriving her of nothing because she will never desire the basic human right to reproduce."[50] For Lord Hailsham: "To talk of the 'basic right' to reproduce of an individual who is not capable of knowing the causal connection between intercourse and childbirth, the nature of pregnancy, what is involved in delivery, unable to form maternal instincts or to care for a child appears . . . wholly to part company with reality."[51] In Dillon L.J.'s opinion the loss of the right would mean "nothing to her."[52] For Lord Oliver the right to reproduce "is of value only if accompanied by the ability to make a choice or indeed to appreciate the need to make one."[53] Is this, one wonders, to be the judicial criterion for the exercise of *all* rights or just the right to reproduce? Generalised, Lord Oliver's reasoning would have some very strange consequences, to which reference will be made subsequently.

That sterilisation was a recourse of "last resort" stressed both in the Court of Appeal (by Dillon and Stephen Brown L.JJ.) and in the House of Lords, most especially in Lord Oliver's speech. The fact that a sterilisation operation is irreversible concerned these but they saw it as the "least detrimental alternative."[54] Lord Oliver stressed that the necessity for the course proposed ha[d] been exhaustively considered by the Official Solicitor on the minor' behalf."[55] The only alternative was the administration daily in pill form of progestogen. Lord Oliver compared the two courses of action. "Of the two possible courses, the one proposed [*i.e.* sterilisation] is safe, certain but irreversible, the other speculative, possibly damaging and requiring discipline over a period of many years from one of the most limited intellectual capacity."[56] His Lordship saw only one way out of this dilemma. "The danger to which she is exposed and the speculative nature of the alternative proposed are such that, on any footing, the risk is not one which should properly be taken by the court."

The Lords were also at pains to point out that their authorisation of a sterilisation was motivated solely by consideration for her welfare and not by any ulterior purposes. She was being treated, in other words, as a person and not as a means to other persons' ends. Thus Lord Hailsham turned roundly on critics who asserted that there might be other considerations when he said: "There is no issue of public policy ... which can conceivably be taken into account, least of all ... any question of eugenics."[57] Lord Oliver was equally forthright and both he and Lord Bridge were insistent that the convenience of Jeanette's carers played no part in their decision-making process.

The Lords were also critical of attempts to draw a distinction between therapeutic and non-therapeutic sterilisations (or presumably medical treatment more generally). The distinction was first drawn by Heilbron J. in *Re D.* in 1975. The learned judge ruled that a decision to carry out a sterilisation for non-therapeutic sterilisations (or presumably medical treatment more generally) was not solely within a doctor's clinical judgment.[58] If this meant that the decision to sterilise a child for therapeutic purposes did lay within exclusive clinical competence, it is a statement that cannot be accepted and, after *Re B.*, for reasons that will become apparent, can no longer represent the law (if it ever did). Heilbron J.'s statement also left open the whole question as to how the therapeutic and non-therapeutic were to be distinguished: on what side of the line did vaccination fall, particularly in controversial cases such as whooping cough? Is circumcision therapeutic or non-therapeutic? The questions are endless.[59]

The distinction assumed importance once again with the judgment in the Canadian Supreme Court of La Forest J. On the facts the learned judge found that "there is no evidence to indicate that failure to perform the operation would have any detrimental effect on Eve's physical or mental health. The purposes of the operation . . . are to protect her from possible trauma in giving birth and from the assumed difficulties she would have in fulfilling her duties as a parent . . . (and) to relieve her of the hygienic tasks associated with menstruation."[60] The judge noted that "the justifications advanced are the ones commonly proposed in support of non-therapeutic sterilization."[61] After examining these justifications (using data culled from the Canadian Law Reform Commission report on Sterilisation) he concluded: "The grave intrusion on a person's rights and the certain physical damage that ensues from non-therapeutic sterilization without consent, when compared to the highly questionable advantages that can result from it, have persuaded me that it can never safely be determined that such a procedure is for the benefit of that person. Accordingly, the procedure should never be authorised for non-therapeutic purposes under *parens patriae* jurisdiction."[62]

Lord Hailsham found La Forest J.'s conclusion "totally unconvincing and in startling contradiction to the welfare principle."[63] The distinction between "therapeutic" and "non-therapeutic" (in the context of this operation) he castigated as "totally meaningless, and, if meaningful, quite irrelevant to the correct application of the welfare principle,"[64] Lord Bridge also thought the distinction diverted "attention from the true issue: namely what was best for Jeanette."[65] He had no intention of indulging in "arid semantic debate" as to where the line was to be drawn between "therapeutic" and "non-therapeutic." But judges indulge in semantic debates all the time and much can hinge on which side of the line the facts of a case are deemed to fall.[66] Are the debates "arid" only where the judges are unprepared to participate in them? Lord Oliver thought the description of the proposed operation in *Re D.* as "non-therapeutic" "apt enough in that case"[67] but nevertheless rejected the distinction in the context of the case he was deciding. It seemed to him 'entirely immaterial whether measures undertaken for the protection against future and foreseeable injury are properly described as "therapeutic." '[68] The real reason, he insisted, was only whether they were for Jeanette's welfare and benefit.

Perhaps the most positive thing to emerge from this sad litigation is to be found in the judgment of Dillon L.J. and in Lord Templeman's speech. Dillon L.J. ruled that neither parents nor a local authority with parental rights could consent to a sterilisation of a minor and that the leave of the Court in wardship proceedings was an essential pre-condition to such an operation taking place.[69] Lord Templeman agreed and added that a doctor performing a sterilisation operation " with the consent of the parents might still be liable in criminal, civil or professional proceedings."[70] His reason was the absence of "a more satisfactory tribunal or a more satisfactory method of reaching a decision."[71] Neither Dillon L.J. nor Lord Templeman said anything to suggest that this ruling applied only to non-therapeutic sterilisations. It must, therefore, be taken to apply to all sterilisations of minors. It is perhaps a pity that the other law lords did not give their express support to Lord Templeman's remarks.[72]

The reason for the rather unseemly haste with which the Jeanette litigation was rushed to a conclusion was the proximity of it to her eighteenth birthday. This raises the question of involuntary sterilisations of mentally handicapped adults. Clearly, they cannot give informed consent,[73] but can anyone give consent on their behalf? This was not a matter upon which the courts had to pronounce and, of course, anything said by them in the course of the Jeanette litigation is strictly *obiter dictum*. Nevertheless, two of the law lords did direct their attention to the question. Lord Hailsham contented himself with referring to the contrast of views in Hoggett[74] and Halsbury[75] and concluded that "whether residual *parens patriae* jurisdiction remains in the High Court after majority"[76] is in doubt. He added that "in twelve months time it would be doubtful . . . what legal courses would be open."[77] Lord Oliver was "prepared to assume" that the *parens patriae* jurisdic-tion did not come to an end when the mentally handicapped person reached the age of majority. He was not, however, prepared to give a ruling in the absence of the much fuller argument which might have been available had a final ruling not been deemed urgent. This reluctance to express an opinion, though predictable, is somewhat unfortunate. It was inevitable that the issue would have to be raised in further litigation and this has, indeed already happened. Not once, but three times.[78]

For the sake of brevity (and to avoid overlap with Brenda Hoggett's paper),[79] I will make a few remarks only about one of these cases. *T* v. *T*[80] concerned the sterilisation of (and an abortion for) a severely mentally handicapped adult. Her mother asked Wood J. for a declaration that the relevant operations without the patient's consent would not constitute an illegal act. T's mental age was even less than Jeanette's. There was no doubt that the abortion sought would satisfy the test in section 1 of the Abortion Act 1967, it being necessary to protect the health of the mother. Was there anyone who could consent on her behalf? It was held that, in the absence of any residual power of *parens patriae* in the court, there was no one who could consent on her behalf. Wood J. concluded that where there is no one who can (or ever will be able to) give consent, a medical adviser is justified in taking such steps as good medical practice demands. He accordingly declared that the operations sought would not be tortious acts merely because of the absence of consent.[81] There is some irony in this ruling for, if it is correct, it becomes easier to sterilise a mentally handicapped adult than a mentally handicapped child: the former rests upon good medical practice, whereas the latter requires judicial intervention. In other words, the haste in Jeanette's case was unnecessary, for upon majority she could have been sterilised without any litigation at all. It is surprising the *T* v. *T* has been subjected to almost no criticism at all.

The issues in *T* v. *T* call to mind both the notorious *Sparkman* case in the United States[82] and *Re Eve*. In *Sparkman* v. *McFarlin* the judge who authorised the sterilisation of a 15 year old girl, said by her mother to be "somewhat retarded," and the doctors who carried out the operation, were sued some years later by the girl and her husband. The US Court of Appeals for the Seventh Circuit held that the action of the judge had no basis in either law (the Indiana statute not being applicable) or equity, and was therefore taken without jurisdiction. The facts of the case defy belief: not only were the girl's interests not independently represented, but she was told the operation was to remove her appendix. The Supreme Court in *Stump* v. *Sparkman* reversed the ruling that the judge had forfeited his immunity. One result of this was that courts subsequently found their jurisdiction to authorise sterilisations in equity, when they could not ground it in a statutory scheme. "Equity" is the functional equivalent of *parens patriae* jurisdiction. The closest we get to a statute is our mental health legislation. But this does not cover the situations envisaged either in Jeanette's case or *T* v. *T* : the compulsory procedures in the Mental Health Act 1983 do not apply.[83] *Parens patriae* jurisdiction over mentally handicapped adults does not seem to have survived the Mental Health Act of 1959, though clearly it could be revived by prerogative action. The question therefore arises as to whether

Wood J. (or the judges involved in the other cases) had jurisdiction to make a declaration. They almost certainly had none in law (the Mental Health Act) and, despite Lord Oliver's remarks in *Re B.*, probably none in "equity" (*parens patriae*). In other words, Wood J. almost certainly lacked the jurisdiction to give the declarations as, of course, did the judges in the other two recent cases. The implications of this are intriguing, raising as they do the authority of a declaration seemingly *ultra vires* and the liability of a judge for the consequences of an act so authorised. But since the judges are undoubtedly immune from actions taken in a judicial capacity,[84] a more serious question to which to direct attention is: how is the gap in the law to be plugged?

The choice is between resurrecting the prerogative power of the Crown and giving the Family Division (or a Family Court) *parens patriae* jurisdiction over the lives ("the custody of the body," as Sir Edward Coke put it in *Beverley's* case[85]) of mentally handicapped adults along the lines of wardship (though as *parens patriae* jurisdiction the case of the mentally handicapped long antedates that of children) and a new statutory formula. I think the latter preferable in the light of the Jeanette saga but it needs to be said that the Canadian Supreme Court coped perfectly adequately with *parens patriae* in *Re Eve*, where the Court held that wardship cases were a "solid guide"[86] to the exercise of *parens patriae* power even in the case of adults. That such power is still vested in Canadian courts when it does not in those in England is the result of differences in statutory law in the last hundred years.

"Jeanette": An Assessment

Any assessment of *Re B.* must use the Canadian Supreme Court decision of *Re Eve* as a critical guide. *Re Eve* was not picked up by those involved in *Re B.* until after the furore caused by the Court of Appeal decision, and insufficient attention was given to it by the House of Lords. Of course, the facts of the two cases are different. Jeanette is severely mentally handicapped, whereas Eve is described as "at least mildly to moderately retarded."[87] We are not (wisely) told her mental age. She is said to suffer from extreme expressive aphasia and to be attracted to, and attractive to, men. Though thought to be able to carry out the mechanical duties of a mother, she was said to be incapable of being a mother in any other sense. The Canadian Supreme Court refused to authorise Eve's sterilisation. Its reasons for doing so are set out in one, very full, well-argued and well-documented judgment. It contains copious reference to periodical literature and, with the assistance of the Canadian Law Reform Commission, an awareness of the research results of those who have studied mental retardation. The court was helped in its deliberations by the participation of several *amici curiae*, who presented the view of interested third parties, enabling it to benefit from the widest range of arguments. It also spent 16 months pondering its judgment. By contrast the House of Lords barely reserved judgment.[88] There were, of course, no *amici curiae*. The speeches are thin. The only judge with Family Division experience declined to give a judgment. The Supreme Court in Canada was honest enough to acknowledge that "judges are generally ill-informed about many of the factors relevant to a wise decision in this difficult area . . . ."[89] *A fortiori*, we can only assume such ignorance in our judiciary, though there is no similar acknowledgment.

The Canadian Supreme Court's decision can best be summarised in one short passage from La Forest J.'s judgment, which has already been quoted.[90] It will be remembered that what he rejected was non-therapeutic sterilisation. The Court, however, agreed that sterilisation might sometimes be necessary and lawful as "treatment of a serious malady."[91] But in the view of the Canadian Supreme Court it was difficult "to imagine a case in which non-therapeutic sterilization could possibly be of benefit to the person on behalf of whom a court purports to act, let alone one in which that procedure is necessary in his or her best interest."[92] La Forest J. was also concerned that any error could not be corrected subsequently. He was aware of the contingency that "nature or the advances of science"[93] might ameliorate Eve's situation. He concluded: "The irreversible and serious intrusion on the basic rights of the individual is simply too great to allow a court to act on the basis of possible advantages which, from the standpoint of the individual, are highly debatable."[94]

It is difficult not to be impressed by both the scholarship and humanity of La Forest J.'s judgment. By contrast the Lords' speeches are shoddy and their compassion unconvincing. I believe the Lords' reasoning was wrong and its conclusion dubious. Why?

(a) *"Best interests" reconsidered*

The core of their decision is that it was for Jeanette's welfare and in her best interests that she be sterilised. To the question what is meant by "best interests," the Lords give only a partial answer. They lay down no guidelines, thus leaving considerable latitude to lower courts and ultimately doctors and others concerned with the care of the mentally handicapped. This is unfortunate because the concept itself is indeterminate, speculative and value-laden. That we have used it, often unthinkingly, in other areas, does not excuse the Lords. We can probably never determine what is a child's best interests,[95] but this should not obstruct us from trying. First, we need information. Secondly, we need predictive ability, to be able to assess the probability of various outcomes and evaluate the advantages and disadvantages of each. Thirdly, we have to admit that our choice will be informed by values: we must be clear what these values are and be prepared to justify our choice of them.

Of these problems the first is the easiest to surmount. We must assume that the Lords were in possession of most of the facts about Jeanette, unlike, for example, the US Supreme Court when it considered Carrie Buck. She was independently represented and the case against sterilisation and in favour of alternative contraceptive measures was put. It is true that alternative forms of contraception have limitations, including some not mentioned in the Lords' speeches (for example with the IUD that of pelvic infection and the risk of expulsion and thus pregnancy). But the assumption was that Jeanette was fertile: the majority of those with severe mental handicap do not have effective fertility.[96] Pregnancy amongst the severely mentally handicapped is extremely rare. According to a letter in the *British Medical Journal* in 1980, perhaps only a score of women with Down's Syndrome had had babies (and only one of these was under 16).[97] How many sterilisations are we prepared to tolerate to save one mentally handicapped woman becoming pregnant? It may be necessary to carry out hundreds of sterilisations to avoid one pregnancy.

If it was really unlikely that Jeanette would become pregnant, was sterilisation the right answer? If she understood as little as the law report seems to indicate, she certainly needed (and needs) protection, in particular from exploitation. It is noticeable how many parents of mentally handicapped daughters complain about their daughters being "raped" by employees of institutions, for example, drivers employed to take them back and forth.[98] One right that the mentally handicapped undoubtedly have is the right not to be sexually abused.[99] Sterilisation does nothing to protect them from sexual exploitation. Saner employment policies (for example the employment of female drivers) and better sex education[1] might achieve rather more.

Once in possession of the "facts," the decision-maker has still got to predict what the probable results of alternative outcomes are. The problem is, as Mnookin observed,[2] that "present-day knowledge about human behaviour provides no basis for the kind

of individualised predictions required by the best-interests standard." There are competing theories of human behaviour related
to different conceptions of human nature and, of course, no
consensus as to which, if any, of these views is the correct one.
Even if there were a right answer, it is difficult to see how it could
be a reliable guide to predict what is likely to happen to a
particular child. But if this applies to "normal" persons, how much
more so is it pertinent to the mentally handicapped? We cannot
even agree on what constitutes mental retardation. A common
interpretation uses a below 70 Intelligence Quotient as a cut-off
point but this would put over two per cent. of the population (or
one million people) into the broad category of mental handicap.
There are any number of different models of mental retardation
and explanations as to its aetiology.[3] Much therefore depends on
interpretation so that prediction itself is heavily dependent on the
model adopted. This must be kept in mind when decisions to
remove a mentally handicapped person's rights are under consideration. Diana Meyers puts this well. She writes: "Because
diagnostic procedures are notoriously fallible and because the
mistaken denial of a person's inalienable rights can be catastrophic, it is necessary to adopt a conservative policy requiring
irrefragable proof of irremediable moral incompetence before an
individual's inalienable rights can be denied."[4] Thus, she indicates, "the protection of inalienable rights extends to many
humans who may never engage in moral relations."[5] And she adds
that "though it is only accidental if all humans qualify for
inalienable rights, few humans will ever be rightfully deprived of
the protection these rights afford."[6] Meyers is not referring to the
right to reproduce (to which right I will return) but her remarks
about diagnostic procedures are very apposite to Jeanette's case.
How can we be certain that Jeanette will not develop? To what
extent is her lack of development due to her total life history? Why
is it, as Zigler points out, that "in the case of the retarded
individual, we seem all too ready to believe that a cognitive
deficiency makes one impervious to those environmental events
known to be central in the genesis of the personality of individuals
of normal intellect?"[7] We know that Jeanette has a mental age of
five or six (whatever that might mean) but do we know what her
mental age would be if she had not had such a depriving and
atypical social history? What has been the effect on her intelligence of constant experiences of failure? It is possible to improve
the behaviour of the retarded through manipulation of environmental events. The danger with decisions like that in Jeanette is
that it is so much easier to avert the supposed danger by sterilising

than to put time, effort and commitment into education, training, counselling and assistance of the mentally handicapped. Their sexual needs and their sexual rights can easily be steamrollered in the name of convenience. Whatever the Lords may say, it was convenient (or "practical" in the language of the reform school administrator) to sterilise Jeanette. It was only in her best interests in so far as these coincided with the best interests of those whose task it was to care for her.

This leads me to the question of values. Much has already been said about this. But a few more remarks are in order. How is utility to be determined? Should best interests be looked at from a long-term or a short-term perspective? How high in the scale of values does physical integrity come? Are we concerned with Jeanette's welfare now or when she is 25 or 50? Supposing Jeanette (or someone in her position) were to be capable of improvement: should the judge in some Rawlsian way decide as the matured handicapped person looking back would have wanted?[8] And what aspect of "welfare" are we emphasising? Is Jeanette better off now? Can we actually answer that question? Can a judge, or five elderly male judges, answer it? It may well be that if sterilisation decisions are to be taken (and I do not rule them out completely) that a court is the most appropriate place to go (though not necessarily one as presently constituted). But more thought than is currently given should be devoted to how such cases are prepared. The details of this lie beyond the scope of this article, but the idea of an inter-disciplinary Ethics Committee as part of a reproductive health clinic for persons with mental handicap, as described by Elkins *et al* in a recent *Hastings Center Report*, is both patient-centred and reflects an awareness of informed societal views.[9] It would be valuable to see such an initiative pursued in this country.

(b) *A right to reproduce?*
It was Heilbron J. in *Re D*. who said that sterilisation (in that case) would deprive a woman of a basic human right, the right to reproduce. In *Re B*., the judges did not deny that the right to reproduce existed, but they held that it meant "nothing" to Jeanette (Bush J., Dillon L.J.) or she couldn't exercise it (Lord Bridge) or the right was of value only if accompanied by the ability to make a choice, of which in Jeanette's case there was no question (Lord Oliver). Discussion of the right to reproduce raises a number of questions.

First, does the right to reproduce exist? Two published articles on the question come to different conclusions. Kingdom,[10] who tells us that "appealing to the right to reproduce is a liability in feminist politics and an obstacle to the development of social policy," concludes there is no right as such to reproduce. She reaches her conclusion after analysing *Re D*. "If," she says, "the possibility of a right to reproduce is dependent on a judgment about the presence or absence of medical grounds for sterilisation" (as it would be if the therapeutic/non-therapeutic distinction is accepted), "then there is no clear basis for ascribing this right to an individual."[11] McLean, on the other hand, believes there is a right to reproduce, though, with both its extent and exercise limited, she has to conclude it is not a "general" right.[12] Gillon's view is similar: he writes of a general prima facie right "not to be stopped."[13] Wald,[14] who like Kingdom and McLean quotes the United States Supreme Court in *Eisenstadt* v. *Baird*,[15] asserts that the right to bear children is a "basic civil right of man (*sic*)." Carby-Hall,[16] in a thoughtful unpublished paper, also assumes the existence of a right to reproduce, though as we shall see, holds that Jeanette for one did not possess it.

What none of these thinkers do is attempt to answer the question *why* we have (or do not have) the right in question. Both Kingdom and McLean make the mistake of examining the positive law and drawing their conclusions (which happen to be different) from their interpretation of legal codes. This is a misleading approach. Even if they were to find the right to reproduce embodied in a legal system (or even in all legal systems), it would not follow that a normatively necessary moral requirement had been established. Whether the right to reproduce exists is independent of what Heilbron J. said in *Re D*. or the House of Lords in *Re B*. It depends on moral argument.

The other thinkers, to which reference has been made, tend to assume the existence of the right in some form or other. This is not surprising. It is all too common to do this. Thus, Nozick asserts peremptorily in the Preface to *Anarchy, State and Utopia*: "individuals have rights."[17] Neither he nor Dworkin[18] tries to explain why we have the rights we do. Nor, for that matter, has either of them explained why they have not tried to explain this.

It is not, however, difficult to explain why rights are important. A society without rights would be morally impoverished. Rights are important because, as Bandman has put it, they "enable us to stand with dignity, if necessary to demand what is our due without having to grovel, plead or beg or to express graditude when we are given our due . . . ."[19] In Feinberg's words: "A world with claim-rights is one which all persons, as actual or potential claimants, are dignified objects of respect . . . No amount of love or compassion, or obedience to higher authority, or *noblesse oblige*, can substitute for those values.[20] Given the social history of this century it is not surprising that we should wish to construct a right to reproduce, or that the United Nations Declaration on Human Rights should talk of "the right to marry and found a family."[21]

But we still need a justifying principle. Why do we have the rights we have and do we have the right to reproduce? One common answer links rights with interests. Such a view was implicit in Bentham and Ihering and is found in such contemporary writers as Feinberg[22] and McCloskey.[23] Thus, Feinberg writes that "the sort of beings who can have rights are precisely those who have (or can have) interests."[24] It is an argument often employed by those who believe that animals have rights.[25] It is also one of the arguments employed by Carby-Hall to demonstrate the Jeanette did not have the right to reproduce. She writes: "A being can truly be said to have an interest in x, the subject of a potential right, if and only if x will benefit him in the sense of furthering some or all of his present or future desires."[26] She argues that a necessary condition of possession of a right is at least the capacity to possess the relevant concepts and a desire for that right. Jeanette clearly lacked the former and almost certainly the latter. But is this association of rights and interests justifiable? I think not. What this does not answer is how the having of interests establishes the grounds for having rights. Animals have interests. I have an interest in Middlesex winning the County Cricket Championship. In neither would it make sense to talk of rights. Human beings do not have the same interests. Surely this does not justify an unequal distribution of human rights. I agree with Alan White that "no valid argument can be given either for including or for excluding children, imbeciles (*inter alia*) . . . as holders of rights on the ground that being capable of having a right ensures or necessitates being capable either of having something in one's interest or of being interested in something. Hence, he concludes, "the question whether animals etc. . . . can or cannot have interests, either in the sense of something being in their interest or in the sense of their being interested in something, is irrelevant to the question whether they can have rights . . . ."[27]

Before we pursue the justifying principle any further it may be as well to ponder the Carby-Hall claim. Can it be right that a necessary condition for the possession of a right is the capacity to possess relevant concepts and a desire for the right in question? Carby-Hall is far from being alone in thinking that it is. In *Causing Death and Saving Lives*, Glover puts the case as follows: "Desires do not presuppose words, but they do presuppose concepts. A baby can want to be fed, or be changed, or go to his mother, although he does not speak. Innumerable signs of recognition and pleasure show us that he has these concepts. But a baby cannot want to escape from death any more than he can want to escape the fate of being a chartered accountant when grown up. He has no idea of either."[28] Glover goes on to argue that the autonomy argument is no objection to infanticide. "In killing a baby, someone is overriding the baby's autonomy to no greater extent than he would be if he prevented the mother from coming home that day."[29] Or, in the language of *Re B.*: "In sterilising Jeanette, we are overriding her autonomy to no greater extent than we would be doing if we prevented her seeing her boyfriend this evening (by, for example, arranging for him to be elsewhere)." I do not find this very convincing. The fact that a baby has no awareness of, or desire for, life cannot mean that it does not have a right to life. It may be difficult, if not impossible, to exercise a right if one is unaware of its existence or one lacks the concepts or the desire, but this cannot mean that one lacks the right in question. If the Carby-Hall-Glover line is correct, what are we to do with the comatose patient, why do we strive to keep alive the potential suicide who has ingested an overdose? Surely, White is right when he argues that it is a "misfortune, not a tautology"[30] that certain persons cannot exercise or enjoy, claim or waive their rights.

In what other ways, then, can rights be grounded? There are any number of justifications. I will consider only a few, and only briefly. There is the intuitionist answer found in thinkers ranging from Jefferson[31] to Nozick.[32] But it offers no argument at all and therefore is unlikely to convince those whose intuitions tell them otherwise. It certainly offers little to resolve the sterilisation dilemma.

There are purely formal answers: the argument that all persons ought to be treated alike unless there is a good reason for treating them differently, that, in other words, persons have the right to equal treatment.[33] But what is a "good reason" for treating persons differently? Gender and colour have now been almost universally accepted as indefensible distinctions: age and intelligence have not. The principle looks egalitarian but potentially could undermine egalitarianism. Those who support the Lords' decision in *Re B.* will find differences between Jeanette and the "normal" woman (lesser intelligence and competence, inability to defer gratification, the ease with which she might be led astray) and those who criticise the decision as unwarranted discrimination will argue that she has more in common with "normal" women than separates her from them (similar feelings, drives, desires and so on). Ironically, if this line of argument is pursued, it becomes relatively easy to defend discrimination by the gifted against those of ordinary intelligence.[34]

An appealing argument was put by William Frankena in an important article in 1962.[35] He argued that humans are "capable of enjoying a good life in the sense in which other animals are not . . . it is the fact that all men are similarly capable of enjoying a good life in this sense that justifies the prima facie requirement that they be treated as equals."[36] Though superficially attractive, there are a number of problems with this. It question-begs. Are all persons capable of enjoying a good life? Those who support the decision to sterilise Jeanette will say she was not, so that the prima facie requirement is removed. Frankena's argument also derives an "ought" from an "is" and fails to show how factual similarity justifies the normative obligation which he supports. Nor is it entirely clear why factual similarity should lead to egalitarian treatment: it would be possible to agree that two persons were similar whilst supporting unequal treatment on the grounds that the value of one person's happiness is greater than that of other persons.[37]

Amongst many other arguments those put forward by Hart in his classic article "Are There Any Natural Rights?"[38] and Rawls in *A Theory of Justice* are too well known (as are their faults) to merit any discussion here. But we cannot ignore the argument contained in the United Nations Universal Declaration of Human Rights, because it is commonly invoked in the sterilisation debate. The first article states: "All human beings are born free and equal in dignity and rights." It is not clear what is meant by "dignity" here or whether it adds anything to "rights." But if "dignity" is identified with respect for persons which leads to their being accorded dignity and hence equality of treatment so far as rights are concerned, the argument is advanced considerably.

I believe it is possible to argue, as Melden[39] does, that we have the rights we do because of our status as moral agents, and that we cannot explain what it is to be a moral agent without eventual reference to our rights. But here we come up against the arguments of Neville.[40] He has two arguments in favour of sterilising the mentally handicapped. One (he calls it the "humble" argument) maintains that sterilisation is in their best interests. His arguments here add little to what has already been said and need no further elaboration or comment. He calls his second argument "philosophical." It is an attempt to defend the policy of sterilisation against the Kantian objection that it is wrong because it denies the subjects their proper place in the moral community, treating them as means only and not ends in themselves, and also against the objection that it is wrong for community representatives to carry out a policy of doing violence to particular subjects.

Neville tries to answer both of these objections. He attempts to neutralise the fears of the objectors. Far from treating persons as things, rather than as responsible agents, Neville claims, he admits somewhat paradoxically, that "to refrain from sterilisation is to do them the violence of preventing them from participating in the moral community in one of the most important respects of which they are capable."[41] The characteristics of the moral community he sets out as follows: (i) membership is relative to the capacity for taking moral responsibility; (ii) most capacities for taking moral responsibility need to be developed; "ordinary socialisation" develops most of them; (iii) a "general moral imperative for any community is that its structures and practices foster the development of the capacities for responsible behaviour whenever possible, and avoid hindering that development."[42] He agrees that the idea of a moral community is "an ideal that exists in pure form only in the imagination."[43] He accepts partial membership for children. But as far as the mildly mentally retarded are concerned (and it should be stressed that he is justifying involuntary sterilisation of the mildly retarded), they, unlike children, do not develop in such a way that "emotional maturity" is achieved at the same time as "bodily maturity." The example he gives could come straight from *Re B*. "For instance, the emotional and intellectual capacities to manage conventional birth control methods, to adjust to pregnancy, or to raise children do not develop by the time their physical development and their social peers among unretarded people are ready for sexual activity."[44]

Neville is prepared to admit mildly mentally retarded people as members of the moral community on condition that they meet certain restrictions, the only one of which he mentions is involuntary sterilisation. What kind of a "moral" community is it that can only admit sterilised members of the class of the mildly mentally handicapped? Neville gropes for an analogy and comes up with an "imperfect" one. "Just as people with bad eyesight may be licensed to drive with the restriction that they wear glasses, so mildly mentally retarded people may be required to meet certain restrictions in order to be members of the moral community."[45] The analogy is "imperfect," he believes, because "a person cannot choose to be in or out of the moral community; one is either in the position to be held responsible or one is not."[46] I believe it is imperfect because it is quite fatuous.

Neville does not spell out his reasons for believing the mildly mentally retarded are irresponsible. I suspect what he has in mind is the supposed inability to care for any children parented, with the burden accordingly falling on the state. But fundamental rights cannot justifiably be abrogated merely because respecting them involves the community in expense. Furthermore, the evidence on parenting competence is shaky. Can imcompetence be tested objectively? "Normal" parents may also be deficient. There is "clear injustice" when a parent "adjudged 'normal' is sometimes able to 'get away' with 'a number of defects in parenting capability, whereas the retarded person, simply because he or she is labelled retarded, is liable to the instigation of sterilisation procedures."[47] Our social control apparatus may not reach as intrusively as the American, but we saw earlier this year the battle waged between Wolverhampton Social Services and a mentally handicapped couple over the question as to whether they could keep their child.[48] To indulge in "slippery slope" arguments is dangerous, but so are slippery slopes.

But we must return to moral agency before we reclimb the slope and examine how slippery it is. How fair are we being to the mentally handicapped? The distinction between "normal" persons and the handicapped is often drawn too starkly. How many of us achieve the ideal of "personhood?" It was Dennett[49] who remarked wisely that few humans are persons in the sense that Kant and Rawls seem to require. We can insist an autonomy not because we are "persons" in the ideal sense of being maximally rational reflective agents, but because, as Wikler put it, "with respect to the challenges [we] have fashioned for [our]selves, [we] are nearly on a par with persons."[50] Very few of us, if any, achieve perfect moral insight.

The rights we have we have simply by virtue of being human. The right to reproduce is one of these rights. Involuntary sterilisation, save where it is carried out for exclusively medical reasons, denies an aspect of humanity. Adequate moral systems must recognise these rights and must do all that is feasible to sustain moral agency. Faced with a choice of changing the world or denying the less able (those who have not achieved and who may never achieve moral agency) access to it, Neville goes for the latter solution. It will be clear that I choose the former solution. If this prioritises the civil liberties of all, including the mentally handicapped, in the name of equal liberty for all at the cost of the general welfare, so be it. But the general welfare should not suffer for it is "a public good ... that [society] is infused with a sense of respect for human beings."[51] A good criterion for judging a society is the way it treats its weaker members.[52]

It may be objected at this point that rights are subject to limitations. How we look at this is heavily dependent upon which conception of rights we adopt.[53] We could adopt a conception of rights as a very important interest, weighted as against other calculations. As such it could be knocked off its pedestal by a goal of special urgency: for example, the right to strike may be forfeited during a war-time emergency.[54] We could also give rights (in Rawls' expression) lexical priority.[55] This would promote them above all other considerations and mean that they clearly prevailed over considerations of utility. This model accepts that rights may conflict with each other, in which case the preferred solution is one which maximises the fulfilment of rights and minimises their violations. A third approach defends the notion of absolute rights: it sees rights as the reason for constraints on action by others.[56] There can be few absolute rights.[57] The right not to be sterilised must come close to being one of them. The main objection to absolute rights is that any right must be overridden if the consequences of fulfilling it are sufficiently disastrous, what Nozick calls "catastrophic moral horror."[58] By accepting, as I have done, that involuntary sterilisation can be defended when it is in the mentally handicapped patient's best medical interests, clearly a lesser test than disaster or horror, I am committing myself to the *second* view of rights. On this view, and returning to Jeanette, it was her rights, and not her welfare, which should have been given first and paramount consideration. Only a compelling reason would justify interference and only then if all less restrictive alternatives had been considered and rejected. In my opinion the House of Lords was too easily convinced that a compelling reason existed in Jeanette's case.

(c) *The slippery slope*

I have left the "slippery slope" argument deliberately to last. It assumed an over-weighty profile in the public debates surrounding the sterilisation of Jeanette. It, rather than an appeal to rights, is an argument (or scenario) with which the public can readily identify. This is not surprising given the social history, to which reference has already been made. Nor should the public's fears be ignored. It is all too easy, as an American court indicated, to drift into policies with unfathomed implications.[59] In a "law-and-order" society with more and more intrusive social control,[60] with bio-technology "improving" reproduction all the time,[61] with Nobel prize-winners calling for licensing of parenthood[62] and favouring temporary sterilisation by means of a time-capsule contraceptive reversed upon government approval,[63] it is as well to be wary.

Slippery slope arguments appeal to the dangerous consequences that can flow from the adoption of particular policies. But slippery slope arguments are themselves dangerous if not structured and carefully thought through. The *logical* implications of a decision must be distinguished from their supposed *empirical* consequences.[64] There is no reason to suppose a logical slippery slope unless it is genuinely feared that courts will permit sterilisation when they do not think it is in the interests of the person concerned. This cannot be foreseen as a danger, but, on the other hand, we cannot predict what will come under the umbrella of "best interests." The shift from *Re D.* to *Re B.* shows how easily "best medical interests" have become "best interests" with the obliteration of the therapeutic/non-therapeutic distinction. It should not be forgotten that a leading gynaecologist wrote in the *Journal of Medical Ethics* in 1975 that "from society's point of view it is rational to encourage sterilisation not only of the mentally abnormal but other groups of disadvantaged individuals." He saw this as "the logical endpoint of genetic counselling."[65] But the logical slippery slope should not become a reality if we ensure that the test remains the best interests of the mentally handicapped person and provide adequate mechanisms to defend those interests.

The problem with the empirical slippery slope argument is, as Gillon indicates, that "it can be used against *any* proposal that is capable of misuse."[66] On the other hand, we will know that sterilisation has been used for social control purposes and not just in the Third Reich. Some of us fear the implications for civil liberties of current law and order policies.[67] And a few of us even remember Sir Keith Joseph's speech in 1972.[68] It would be a wise person who could declare for certainty that there is no danger of sterilisation policies being pursued beyond the range intended by the Lords in Jeanette's case. The case for an empirical slippery slope is unproven and unprovable, but I would not rule it out. At the very least the Lords' decision helps to foster an ideology which denies human rights and, in doing so, denies the humanity of an already disadvantaged group of people.

Conclusion

I have criticised the House of Lords for (i) putting what they conceived to be Jeanette's best interests before her rights; for (ii) the way they identified those interests, in particular their refusal to accept that best interests means in this context "best medical interests" and for (iii) giving too little consideration to Jeanette's rights, and not taking them seriously. Further, on best interests they offer little guidance, thus creating enormous latitude for subsequent decision-makers. The only positive things to emerge from this sad litigation are the rejection (once again) of parental rights and clinical freedom (in particular in Lord Templeman's speech) and, most importantly, the opportunity the saga offers us to rethink the rights of the mentally handicapped.[69] If something positive comes out of a rethink, then Jeanette will not have suffered in vain.

Notes

[1] *Re Adoption Application 212/86*, [1987] 2 F.L.R. 291; *Re P.* [1978] 2 F.L.R. 421.
[2] *C.* v. *S.* [1987] 1 All E.R. 1230.
[3] *D.* v. *Berkshire C.C.* [1987] 1 All E.R. 20.
[4] *R.* v. *Ethical Committee of St Mary's Hospital, ex p. Harriott, The Independent,* October 27, 1987.
[5] *Re B.* [1987] 2 All E.R. 206.
[6] *The Daily Telegraph*, April 16, 1987.
[7] March 17, 1987.
[8] Raanan Gillon, "On Sterilising Severely Mentally Handicapped People," (1987) 13 J. Med. Ethics 59 at 61.
[9] Another good illustration is the *Arthur* case which Raanan Gillon uses as the theme of his *Philosophical Medical Ethics*, Wiley, 1986.
[10] *Op. cit.*, note 5, p. 213.
[11] (1986) 31 D.L.R. (4th ed.) 1, 29.
[12] Quoted in Moya Woodside, *Sterilisation In North Carolina*, Univ. of N. Carolina Press, 1950, p. 81. See Also E.S. Gosney and P. Popenol, *Sterilisation for Human Betterment*, MacMillan, 1930.
[13] The founder of the eugenics movement was Sir Francis Galton. As an undergraduate at U.C.L. most of my lectures took place in the Eugenics Theatre. The term was coined in the 1880's.
[14] Another failed in Pennsylvania in 1904. It passed the legislature but was vetoed by the Governor.
[15] See (eds.) R. Macklin and W. Gaylin, *Mental Retardation and Sterilisation*, Plenum Press, 1981, pp. 64–65.
[16] 274 U.S. 200 (1927).
[17] Holmes, as a jurist, viewed law from the "standpoint" of the "bad man" ("The Path of the Law" (1897) 10 Harv. L. Rev. 457–478).
[18] *Op. cit.*, note 16, p. 207. An interesting postscript on the case is S.J. Gould, *The Mismeasure of Man*, Penguin, 1984, pp. 335–336.
[19] [1954] 3 All E.R. 59. See my comment in *Lord Denning: The Judge and the Law* (eds. J.L. Jowell and J.P.W.B. McAuslan), Sweet and Maxwell, 1984, pp. 111–112.
[20] Herbert Spencer in *Social Statics* (1850) argued that the individual should be allowed to make avoidable fatal mistakes because in this way the inefficient and the stupid would be eliminated and the human species improved.
[21] *Skinner* v. *Oklahoma* 316 U.S. 535 (1942); *Relf* v. *Weinberger* 372 F. Supp. 1196

(1974); *Cook* v. *State* 495 P. 2d. 768 (1972); *North Carolina Assn. for Retarded Children* v. *North Carolina* 420 F. Supp. 451 (1976). See, further, M. Bayles in *op. cit.*, note 13, Chap. 11, and J.H. Landman, *Human Sterilisation*, MacMillan, 1932 (useful especially for the laws and legal decisions, as well as the history generally).

22 "Positive" eugenics has, however, come into fashion among the "Moral Right," see for example, the proposals in R.K. Graham, *The Future of Man*, Foundation for the Advancement of Man, 1981. An excellent critique in G. Corea, *The Mother Machine*, Harper and Row, 1985, Chap. 1.

23 420 F. Supp. 451 (1976).

24 *Ibid.* p. 455.

25 *Ibid.* p. 456.

26 *Ibid.* p. 454.

27 This figure is quoted in D. Meyers, *The Human Body and the Law*, (1971) Edinburgh University Press, p. 29. Of these 27,917 were sterilised on grounds of mental illness and 32,374 on grounds of mental deficiency.

28 "Voluntary Sterilization: Counseling and Informed Consent" in *Proceedings of the 5th World Congress on Medical Law*, 1979, p. 64.

29 See Jane Mercer, *Labeling the Mentally Retarded*, (1973) Univ. of California Press. On the psychological impact see P. Roos, (1975) *Law and Psychology Review* 45–56.

30 It is estimated that there were 300,000 victims.

31 See F. Pfafflin and J. Gross (1982) 5 Int. J. of Law and Psychiatry 419–423.

32 Another recent example is El Salvador.

33 [1976] 1 All E.R. 326.

34 *Hansard*, H.C. vol. 894, col. 629, 635, (June 25, 1975).

35 September 1, 1975.

36 (1975) 1 J. Med. Ethics 161.

37 January 14, 1976.

38 *Op. cit.*, note 33, p. 333.

39 *The Independent*, March 21, 1987.

40 See (1975) 1 J. Med. Ethics, 163.

41 2nd ed., 1987, p. 62.

42 *Idem.*

43 *Op. cit.*, note. 5, p. 219.

44 *Ibid.* p. 209.

45 Guardianship of Minors Act 1971, s.1 and *J.* v. *C.* [1970] A.C. 668 at 710 *per* Lord MacDermott.

46 *Per* Dunn J. in *Re D.* [1977] Fam. 158 at 163.

47 For example, *Re X.* [1975] Fam. 47; *S.* v. *McC.* [1972] A.C. 24. Lord Hailsham's own reasoning in *Richards* v. *Richards* [1984] A.C. 174 (not a wardship case) should also not be ignored.

48 *Op. cit.*, note 5, p. 215.

49 *Op. cit.*, note 33, p. 332.

50 *Op. cit.*, note 5, p. 208.

51 *Ibid.* p. 213.

52 *Ibid.* p. 210.

53 *Ibid.* p. 219.

54 The term (in another context) belongs to Goldstein, Freud and Solnit, *Beyond the Best Interests of the Child*, Free Press, 1973, pp. 53–64.

55 *Op. cit.*, note 5, p. 217.

56 *Ibid.* p. 218.

57 *Ibid.* p. 212.

[58] *Op. cit.*, note 33, p. 335. *Cf.* Wood J. in *Re T* (*post*, p. 65).

[59] See N. Lowe and R. White, *Wards of Court* (2nd ed., 1986), Barry Rose, pp.88–89.

[60] *Op. cit.*, note. 11, pp. 30–31

[61] *Ibid.* p. 31.

[62] *Ibid.* p. 32.

[63] *Op. cit.*, note 5, p. 213.

[64] *Idem.*

[65] *Ibid.* p. 214.

[66] A point made especially well by Glanville Williams, "Language and the Law" (1945) 61 L.Q.R. 183–185.

[67] *Op. cit.*, note. 5, p. 219.

[68] *Idem.*

[69] *Ibid.* pp. 210–211.

[70] *Ibid.* p. 214.

[71] *Ibid.* p. 215.

[72] Particularly, in the light of Wood J.'s judgment in *T* v. *T* ([1988] 2 W.L.R. 189) that, where *an adult* was concerned, "a medical adviser is justified in taking such steps as good medical practice demands." (p. 204).

[73] A useful article (on U.S. law) is G.S. Neuwirth *et al*, "Capacity, Competence, Current: Voluntary Sterilization of the Mentally Retarded" (1975) 6 Columbia Human Rights. R. 451.

[74] *Mental Health Law*, 2nd ed. 1984, p. 203.

[75] *Laws of England* vol. 8, 4th ed. 1974, para. 901, note 6.

[76] *Op. cit.*, note. 5, p. 212.

[77] *Ibid.* p. 218.

[78] The first (by Latey J. on May 14, 1987) is unreported; the second (*Re X*), a decision of Reeve J. is reported in *The Times*, June 4, 1987. For the third see below note 80.

[79] *Post*, p. 85.

[80] [1988] 2 W.L.R. 189.

[81] Of course, he did not (and could not) declare that they would not be criminal acts.

[82] 532 F. 2d 172 (1977), reversed in *Stump* v. *Sparkman.* (1978) 435 U.S. 349.

[83] The 1983 Act framework embraces only medical treatment for mental disorders; it does not apply to treatment for physical disorders, or operations of a non-therapeutic nature such as a vasectomy or an abortion.

[84] *Scott* v. *Stansfield* (1868) L.R. 3 Ex. 220, 223.

[85] (1603) 4 Co. Rep. 123b, at 126a, 126b (76 E.R. 1118, 1124).

[86] *Op. cit.*, note 11, p. 14.

[87] *Ibid.* p. 4. *per* McQuaid J. (in lower court).

[88] Lord Brandon of Oakbrook.

[89] *Op. cit.*, note 11, p. 32.

[90] *Ante*, p. 63.

[91] *Op. cit.*, note 11, p. 34.

[92] *Ibid.* p. 32.

[93] *Idem.*

[94] *Idem.*

[95] On indeterminacy see R. Mnookin, *In the Interest of Children*, W.H. Freeman, 1985 particularly pp. 16–24.

[96] See the letters by D. Chakrabanti and B. Kirman in 281 *British Medical Journal* 1281–1282 (1980).

[97] By B. Kirman (see note 96), and also in Symposium on "Child Sterilisation" in (1975) 1 J. Med. Ethics 163–167.

82   *Sterilising the Mentally Handicapped*

This point was forcefully made on the BBC TV "Kilroy" programme.
See J. Ennew, *The Sexual Exploitation of Children*, Polity Press. 1986.
¹ See in R. Ives, B. Franklin (ed.), *The Rights of Children*, Blackwell, 1986 Chap.7.
² "Child-Custody Adjudication: Judicial Functions in the Face of Indeterminacy," (1975) 39 *Law and Contemporary Problems* 226 at 258.
³ There are over 200 known causes of mental retardation. A good account is R.W. Conley, *The Economics of Mental Retardation*, The Johns Hopkins Press, 1973, Chaps. II & III.
⁴ *Inalienable Rights: A Defence*, Columbia U.P. 1985, p. 141.
⁵ *Idem.*
⁶ *Idem.*
⁷ "The Retarded Child As A Whole Person" in (ed.) D.R. Routh, *The Experimental Psychology of Mental Retardation*, Aldine, 1973, p. 231 at 237.
⁸ On Rawls see *A Theory of Justice*, Harvard University Press 1971. See also M.D.A. Freeman "Taking Children's Right Seriously" in *Children and Society* vol. 1 no. 4, p. 299 (1988).
⁹ (1986) Hastings Center Report vol. 16 (3), pp. 20–22.
¹⁰ "The Right to Reproduce" in (ed.) M. Ockleton, *Medicine, Ethics and Law*, p. 54.
¹¹ *Ibid.* p. 57.
¹² "The Right to Reproduce" in T. Campbell *et al*, *Human Rights*, Blackwell, 1986, p. 99, 112.
¹³ *Op. cit.*, note 8 (1st series), p. 60.
¹⁴ "Basic Personal and Civil Rights" in (ed.) M. Kindred *et al*, *The Mentally Retarded Citizen and the Law*, Free Press, 1976, p. 3 at 11.
¹⁵ 405 U.S. 438 (1972). "If the right to privacy means anything, it is the right of the individual, married or single, to be free from unwarranted governmental intrusion into matters so fundamentally affecting a person as the decision whether to beget or bear a child." (p. 453).
¹⁶ "The Right to Reproduce." I am grateful to Felicity Carby-Hall, a Ph.D. student of mine, for giving me the permission to comment upon her work in this way, somewhat exceeding normal tutorial licence!
¹⁷ Basic Books, 1974, p. ix.
¹⁸ In *Taking Rights Seriously*, Duckworth, 1978 (revised ed.).
¹⁹ "Do Children Have Any Natural Rights?" (1973) *Proceedings of 29th Annual Meeting of Philosophy of Education Society*, p. 234 at 236.
²⁰ "Duties, Rights and Claims" (1966) 3 Amer. Phil. Q. 137.
²¹ Art. 16(1).
²² "The Nature and Value of Rights" (1970) Journal of Value Inquiry 243–260.
²³ "Rights" (1965) 15 Phil. Q. 115–127. In a later article he holds that persons have a prima facie right to the satisfaction of needs, (1976) 13 Amer. Phil. Q. 9.
²⁴ *Rights, Justice and the Bounds of Liberty*, (1980), Princeton U.P., p. 167.
²⁵ For example, J. Feinberg (see "The Rights of Animals and Unborn Generations" in W. Blackstone (ed.), *Philosophy and Environment Crisis*, (1974). See also M.A. Warren; "Do Potential People have Moral Rights?" (1977) VII Canadian J. of Phil. 275–89.
²⁶ *Op. cit.*, note 16 (2nd series), p. 18.
²⁷ *Rights*, Clarendon Press, 1984, p. 82.
²⁸ Penguin Books, 1977, p. 158.
²⁹ *Idem.*
³⁰ *Op. cit.*, note 27, p. 90.
³¹ Who held it to be "self-evident" that all humans equally have certain rights. A

good account is C.D. Brown, *Miracle At Philadelphia*, Little Brown, 1966.
[32] *Anarchy, State and Utopia*, Basic Books, 1974.
[33] Ch. Perelman, *The Idea of Justice and the Problem of Argument*, (1963), RKP, pp. 15–16; H.L.A. Hart, *The Concept of Law*, (1961) Clarendon Press, p. 158. *Cf.* R. Dworkin, *op. cit.*, note 117 at 227.
[34] See the arguments of Daniel Wikler, "Paternalism and the Mildly Retarded" (1979) 8 Phil. and Public Affairs 377–392.
[35] "The Concept of Social Justice" in R. Brandt, *Social Justice*, (1962), Prentice-Hall, p. 1.
[36] *Ibid.* p. 19.
[37] *Cf.* G. Vlastos, "Justice and Equality,' in *op. cit.*, note 134, pp. 52–53 (note 45).
[38] (1955) 64 Phil. Review 175.
[39] *Rights and Persons*, O.U.P., 1977.
[40] "Sterilising the Mildly Mentally Retarded Without Their Consent: The Philosophical Arguments" in (eds.) R. Macklin and W. Gaylin, *op. cit.*, note 15, pp. 181–193.
[41] *Ibid.* pp. 190–191.
[42] *Ibid.* p. 186.
[43] *Idem.*
[44] *Ibid.* p. 187.
[45] *Ibid.* p. 189.
[46] *Idem.*
[47] *Op. cit.*, note 15 (1st series), p. 96.
[48] *The Guardian*, July 2, 1987.
[49] "Conditions of Personhood" in A. Rorty (ed.), *The Identities of Persons*, (1976), Univ. of California Press, pp. 175–196.
[50] *Ibid.*
[51] *Per* J. Raz, "Right-Based Moralities" in R.S. Frey (ed.), *Utility and Rights*, (1985) Blackwell, p. 42 at 46–47. See also now *The Morality of Freedom*, (1986) O.U.P. Chap. 8.
[52] *Cf.* Urie Bronfenbrenner, *Two Worlds of Childhood*, (1970) Russell Sage, or B. Blatt, *Exodus from Pandemonium.* (1970), Allyn and Bacon.
[53] See J. Waldron, *Theories of Rights* (1984) O.U.P.
[54] See L.J. MacFarlane, *The Right to Strike*, (1981) Penguin, pp. 127–132.
[55] *A Theory of Justice*, (1971) Harvard University Press, pp. 42–45.
[56] See *op. cit.*, note 152, p. 15.
[57] See Alan Gewirth, *Human Rights*, (1982) Univ. of Chicago Press, Chap. 9.
[58] In *op. cit.*, note 32 (2nd series), at p. 29.
[59] *Relf* v. *Weinbeger* (1974) 372 F. Supp. 1196.
[60] For historical and theoretical insights see S. Cohen and A. Scull, *Social Control and the State*, (1983) Martin Robertson. On contemporary issues see S. Cohen, *Visions of Social Control*, (1985). Polity Press.
[61] M. Stanworth, *Reproductive Technologies*, (1987) Polity Press. G. Corea, *The Mother Machine*, (1985), Harper and Row; R. Arditti (ed.), *Test-Tube Woman*, (1985), Pandora Press.
[62] William Shockley, winner of Nobel Prize for making transistors. See the discussions of his ideas in Corea, *op. cit.*, note 160, pp. 25–27.
[63] These views of Shockley are traced in C. Djerassi, *The Politics of Contraception.*, (1979), W.W. Norton, p. 180. Francis Crick (co-discoverer of the cell's DNA structure) expressed similar views at a CIBA conference in 1963 and reported in G. Wolstenholme (ed.), *Man and His Future*, 1963, Churchill.
[64] And see R. Gillon, *op. cit.*, note 8 (1st series), p. 61.
[65] *Per* M. Brudenell, (1975) 1 J. Med. Ethics 163, 164.

[66] *Op. cit.*, note 8 (1st series), p. 61. On "slippery slopes" generally see B. Williams "Which Slopes are Slippery?" in (ed.) M. Lockwood, *Moral Dilemmas in Modern Medicine*, (1986) Oxford, pp. 126–137.

[67] See M.D.A. Freeman, "Law and Order in 1984" (1984) 37 *Current Legal Problems* 175–231. The Police and Criminal Evidence Act 1984, the Public Order Act 1986, further attacks on the jury and on the press (note the use of civil law injunctions rather than the discredited Official Secrets Act prosecution, where there is a good chance of a jury acquitting), all provide further ammunition for the thesis presented there.

[68] "The Cycle of Deprivation" in (eds.) E. Butterworth and R. Holman, *Social Welfare In Modern Britain*, (1975) Fontana, pp. 387–93 (somewhat retracted in an article on Social Class in *The Guardian*, July 18, 1979.)

[69] See W. Kempton, "Sexual Rights and Responsibilities of the Retarded Person" in *The Social Welfare Forum 1976*, (1977), Columbia U.P., pp. 206–220; B. Gray, "Whose Handicap?" in (ed.) D. Carson, *The Law and the Sexuality of People wih a Mental Handicap*, (1987), University of Southampton, pp. 7–12.

The Royal Prerogative in Relation to the Mentally Disordered: Resurrection, Resuscitation, or Rejection?*

BRENDA HOGGETT

Introduction

In the second edition of *Mental Health Law*, I delivered myself of the view that "we clearly need someone to resurrect the ancient prerogative power of the Crown to protect these patients, along similar lines to the modern development of the prerogative jurisdiction to protect wards of court."[1] In retrospect this seems unwise, both linguistically and substantively. Linguistically, it allowed Lord Hailsham in the course of argument in *Re B. (a minor) (wardship: sterilisation)*[2] to suggest that resuscitation of the unconscious would be more appropriate than resurrection of the dead. In *T* v. *T*[3] Mr. Justice Wood went even further in urging the "speedy restitution" of the jurisdiction, which suggests that some members of the judiciary may well be tempted to regard it as a natural right of which they have been wrongly deprived. My purpose now, therefore, is to consider the present status of that jurisdiction and, more importantly, whether it can and should be revived.

The context of my observations, and of these cases, was medical treatment for adult mentally handicapped people. Where such a person is incapable in law of giving an effective consent to treatment, it is now generally agreed that no other person is automatically entitled to consent on his behalf.[4] It is also agreed that the Mental Health Act 1983 provides no statutory procedure for conferring such a power on any person.

The Act does provide for compulsory admission to and treatment in hospital; but even where the patient is severely mentally handicapped, for long-term measures there must be associated "abnormally aggressive or seriously irresponsible

85

conduct," and in any event the treatment is limited to treatment
for the mental disorder from which the patient is suffering.[5] The
Act also provides for guardianship in the community, but again
only for the same categories of patient, and the guardian has no
power to authorise treatment.[6] These limitations were quite
deliberately inserted in order to remove the general run of
handicapped patients from the ambit of the Act and to restrict the
scope of compulsion within the community. Despite quite a strong
medical lobby in favour of the power to impose treatment without
compulsory admission, the view which prevailed at the time was
that the necessary safeguards would only be effective in a hospital
setting.

Nevertheless, doctors undoubtedly do have some authority to
proceed without consent but the boundaries of this are far
from clear. No one seriously doubts that doctors may proceed
with treatment which is so necessary and urgent that it cannot
reasonably be postponed until a valid consent can be
obtained.[7] The problem has always been to find an acceptable
rationalisation for this. Any doctrine of necessity is highly controversial in both civil and criminal law. The doctrine of
implied consent cannot cater for those cases in which the
patient would not or could not have consented. With an adult
mentally handicapped patient, it may never be possible to
obtain a valid consent. A third possibility has recently been
suggested, undoubtedly *obiter*, by Lord Justice Croom-Johnson
in *Wilson* v. *Pringle*,[8] when adopting the general exception to
the tort and crime of battery put forward by Lord Justice
Robert Goff in *Collins* v. *Wilcock*.[9] This embraces "all physical
contact which is generally acceptable in the ordinary conduct of
every day life." An urgent operation by a casualty surgeon
upon an unconscious patient may well fall into this category.
Sterilisation of a permanently incapable patient is surely a
more difficult case.

Two sorts of justification have been adopted in the recent
cases concerning mentally handicapped women. On one view,
treatment can be given if it is necessary to save life or to
prevent a serious deterioration in physical or mental health, as
seems to have been the view taken by Mr. Justice Latey in a
recent unreported decision[10] and by Mr. Justice Reeve in *Re
X*.[11] On another view, if the patient is unlikely ever to be able
to consent, doctors may proceed with whatever is for the medical benefit of the patient. This is, perhaps surprisingly, the
view taken by Larry Gostin[12] and, most recently, by Mr. Justice Wood in *T* v. *T*:

"I am content to rely on the principle that in these exceptional circumstances where there is no provision in law for consent to be given and therefore there is no one who can give the consent, and where the patient is suffering from such mental abnormality as never to be able to give such consent a medical adviser is justified in taking such steps as good medical practice 'demands' . . . "[12a]

In all three recent cases declarations were granted that an abortion, and in *T* v. *T* a sterilisation, would not be unlawful; these declarations will no doubt be effective to avert any action by or on behalf of the patient for damages, but could not bind a criminal court in the event of a subsequent prosecution.[13]

It is difficult to understand why Mr. Justice Wood should at one and the same time both uphold a wide common law justification for doctors to decide on behalf of the patient and call for the speedy restitution of the courts' jurisdiction to do so. If the doctors can decide, what need have they for the courts' authority, other than perhaps by way of declaration in cases where there is a genuine doubt as to what good medical practice demands? Were the prerogative jurisdiction to be revived, might it not carry the implication that no such steps can be taken without resort to the court? After all, in *Re B.*[14] Lord Templeman went out of his way to say that:

"A court exercising the wardship jurisdiction emanating from the Crown is the only authority which is empowered to authorise such a drastic step as sterilisation after a full and informed investigation. No one has suggested a more satisfactory tribunal or a more satisfactory method of reaching a decision which vitally concerns an individual but also involves principles of law, ethics and medical practice."

The resounding silences of the other judges on this occasion may be significant, but as we shall see later the theoretical justification for this point of view in relation to the mentally handicapped is if anything greater than it is in relation to children.

The issue arose in the context of medical treatment, specifically abortion and sterilisation, but it is in fact part of a much wider debate about the civil status of severely mentally handicapped adults. The United Nations declaration on the rights of mentally retarded persons proclaims that they should enjoy the same rights as other people, to the maximum degree of feasibility, and this must include the right to decide for themselves whenever possible.

If they are unable to do so, or it becomes necessary to restrict or deny their rights, there should be proper legal safeguards. The procedure "must be based on the evaluation of the social capability of the mentally retarded person by qualified experts and must be subject to periodic review and to the right of appeal to higher authorities."[15] These aims are difficult to reconcile with our present mental health legislation, which since 1959 has been avoiding the issue of whether procedures which are necessary to secure the cooperation of an actively protesting patient may sometimes be just as necessary to secure the protection of a patient who is unable to express a view one way or the other.

Wardship: A False Analogy?

At first sight, it would seem surprising if a revival of the prerogative jurisdiction could supply the answer to these problems. The whole history of legislation in the field of mental health has been in the direction of defining the exercise of the prerogative or finding alternatives to it. The attraction today no doubt stems from the analogy with the modern wardship jurisdiction over children, coupled with the sort of absurdity revealed in *Re B*. How could it properly be relevant to such an important decision that if the sterilisation were not performed before the patient reached 18 it might never be performed at all?

However, we should bear in mind that the ancient wardship jurisdiction was also fading away until its remarkable revival after the Second World War.[16] Reasons for its revival included the procedural rationalisation in the Law Reform (Miscellaneous Provisions) Act 1949, legal aid, and the structural rationalisation in the Administration of Justice Act 1970; a profound philosophical change, culminating in the House of Lords' decision in *J. v. C.*[17]; and the increasing sophistication of local authority activities in the protection of children, affording both an alternative means available to the court of exercising its protective jurisdiction and a fertile source of applications to do so. It is only in the last two decades that wardship has developed into the genuinely all-embracing protective jurisdiction which is exemplified by decisions such as *Re D. (a minor) (wardship: sterilisation)*.[18]

Quite apart from the historical distinctions between the two jurisdictions, the analogy between the protection of children and the protection of adult handicapped people can never be exact.

First, the court's jurisdiction over children can arise automatically by reference to the objectively determinable fact of age; a similar automatic jurisdiction does not and cannot apply to the handicapped. Secondly, the court's powers in wardship are there to supplement, override or replace the powers and responsibilities of parents; although the court's powers may be somewhat more extensive, at least in their enforceability, they are operating against a background of existing powers over and responsibilities for the upbringing of children. No such powers and responsibilities can be assumed in respect of adult handicapped people. Thirdly, therefore, if the court does not intervene to take a particular decision about a child, it may generally be assumed that somebody else would be able to do so; depending upon the nature of the decision and the capacities of the child, this may be either the parents or the child himself. As we have already seen, if the adult handicapped person does not himself have the capacity to take the particular decision, there is usually no one who can take it on his behalf. These distinctions may support rather than undermine the case for some protective machinery, but they also suggest that it cannot be quite like the machinery applied to children. A brief, and necessarily preliminary, look at the history of the prerogative in relation to the mentally disordered bears this out.

The Prerogative[19]

The origin of the ancient prerogative can be found in the right of the feudal lord to the wardship of the lands and person of a tenant of unsound mind who was thus unable to render the required services. This right was apparently taken over by the Crown, either by general assent or by statute, towards the end of the reign of Henry III. The existence of the right, now called a prerogative, was recognised in the "statute" *de Praerogativa Regis*, generally cited as 17 Edward II, c. 9 and 10, but thought by Maitland to be a "tract written by some lawyer in the early years of Edward I"[20] although possibly issued on the authority of the King. Whatever it was, it recognised and delimited, rather than created, the prerogatives there set out. It provided one rule for idiots:

> "The King shall have the custody of the lands of natural fools, taking the profits of them without waste or destruction, and shall find them their necessaries, of whose fee soever the lands be holden; and after the death of such idiots he shall render it to the right heirs, so that such idiots shall not aliene, nor their heirs shall be disinherited."

And a different rule for lunatics:

> "The King shall provide when any, that beforetime hath his
> wit and memory happen to fail of his wit, as there are many
> [per lucida intervalla], that their lands and tenements shall be
> safely kept without waste and destruction, and that they and
> their household shall live and be maintained competently with
> the profits of the same, and the residue besides their
> sustentation shall be kept to their use, to be delivered unto
> them when they come to their right mind; so that such lands
> and tenements shall in no wise be aliened; and the King shall
> take nothing to his own use. And if the party die in such
> estate, then the residue shall be distributed for his soul by the
> advice of the ordinary."[21]

Hence while the King was entitled to keep the profits over and
above those needed to maintain the idiot and his family, he had to
account for those of a lunatic. In the eighteenth century,
Blackstone could still list the incomes of idiots' estates as a source
of revenue for the Crown. But he also tells us that this was rarely
abused, because juries usually refused to return a verdict of idiocy
from birth.[22] In practice, therefore, the prerogative over idiots'
property was the same as that over lunatics'. The principal purpose
had long been to protect and preserve the property and the
patient, rather than to secure a benefit for the Crown. The benefit
would normally go to the heir, next of kin or creditors, who were
therefore most likely to invoke the jurisdiction.

There cannot be any serious doubt that the Crown's prerogative
extended to the control of the person as well as the property of the
patient. Lord Coke in *Beverley's* case[23] stated that:

> "Although the statute says *custodiam terrarum* yet the King
> shall have as well the custody of the body and of their goods
> and chattels as of the lands and other hereditaments and as
> well those which he has by purchase as those which he has as
> heir by the common law."

This statement arose in the context of debate as to whether the
prerogative extended to chattels real and personal, but the Crown
undoubtedly asserted the right to have or provide for the custody
of idiots or lunatics,[24] and this was reflected in the common
practice of appointing a committee of the person as well as of the
property, in appropriate cases; statutory recognition of both can
be found, for example in the provisions of the Lunacy Act 1890.[25]

However, while we can be sure that the Crown enjoyed a wide prerogative power to protect the person and property of some mentally incapacitated people, we can be equally sure that there were important limitations. Each of these indicates how different the jurisdiction was, both in its origin and in its developed state, from the jurisdiction over children. First, historically the power was only exercised after the person had been found idiot or lunatic by inquisition. Once upon a time, perhaps, it arose without any such process. But the issue of writs *de idiota* or *de lunatico inquirendo* dates back for almost as long as there is learning on this subject, and a finding after such inquisition appears to have been a *sine qua non* for the exercise of the Crown's powers. The Lord Chancellor issued these writs, upon the appropriate petitions, just as he does any other.[26] They were originally addressed to escheators and Theobald cites numerous statutes regulating the conduct of these matters.[27] Subsequently, the writ was superseded by a Commission under the Great Seal, addressed to five Commissioners. Until 1853, the question was always decided with the help of a jury. Nineteenth century legislation[28] provided for general commissions of enquiry directed at Commissioners, later Masters, in Lunacy, for the issue to be tried by a Judge of the King's Bench in appropriate cases, and for inquisitions to be held without the assistance of a jury unless the alleged lunatic demanded one. The odd instance may be found of Lord Eldon interfering in the affairs of a person who had not been found lunatic by inquisition,[29] but the texts all support the view of Lord Brougham[30] that:

"The lord chancellor as intrusted, by virtue of the king's sign manual, with the care and commitment of the custody of the persons and estates of lunatics, has no jurisdiction to refer it to the master to inquire into the state of mind of lunatics against whom no commission has issued, or to make orders relative to the care of their persons and property and to their maintenance; and although, in certain cases, where the property of persons of unsound mind is too small to bear the expenses of a commission, it is very desirable that the lord chancellor sitting in lunacy should possess such jurisdiction, it can only be conferred by the legislature."

It is significant that later legislation conferred analagous powers over the property of certain other categories of person.[31]

Secondly, once the existence of the Crown's powers had been established by this means, it was necessary for the powers to be delegated by the Crown to some authority which could exercise them on the Crown's behalf. Originally they were given to the Exchequer, as an aspect of tax collection. Once they became more of a duty, they passed to the Lord Chancellor. While the Court of Wards existed, the jurisdiction was generally exercised by that court. Once the court was abolished, in 1660, delegation was almost always to the Lord Chancellor and later to two Lords Justices as well. This delegation was effected by Royal Warrant under the Sign Manual, which was reissued at the beginning of every reign. The jurisdiction cannot therefore be regarded as one which is "inherent" in the High Court or in any individual.

Thirdly, by virtue of this delegation, the Chancellor or other delegate would appoint and control a committee of the person or of the estate of the patient or of both. Statutes during the nineteenth century provided several other express powers. The jurisdiction in lunacy, however, was quite different from the ordinary jurisdiction of the Court of Chancery. As was said in *Beall* v. *Smith*:[32]

> "Unsoundness of mind gives the Court of Chancery no jurisdiction whatever. It is not like infancy in that respect. The Court of Chancery is by law the guardian of infants whom it makes its wards. The Court of Chancery is not the curator either of the person or the estate of a person *non compos mentis*, whom it does not, and cannot make its ward. . . ."

Once again, as with the inquisition, there are indications that some judges were prepared to assert a wider Chancery jurisdiction over lunatics "not so found."[33] They are roundly taken to task in the texts[34] which are supported by no less a modern authority than Mr. Justice Megarry, in *Re K.'s Settlement Trusts*.[35] After an extensive review of the authorities, he decided that Chancery would only intervene if there was money in court or some other proceeding giving the court control over the property,[36] and even then only if the estate was small and no proceedings in lunacy were likely. It seems clear, therefore, that an independent Chancery jurisdiction does not exist.

The many statutory interventions to improve the exercise of the prerogative powers were consolidated by the Lunacy Act 1890. Part IV of that Act almost has the appearance of a complete code for the management of the property of mentally disordered persons, but it does still assume the existence of prerogative powers, at least in relation to people found lunatic by inquisition. In *Re Sefton*[37] the court exercised a power of sale, which could not be found in the 1890 Act but was justified by reference to the main purpose of *praerogativa regis* in protecting the value of the lunatic's estate; the Earl of Sefton had, however, already been found lunatic by inquisition.

These provisions should be distinguished from the other powers which were also consolidated in that Act (and the similar powers created in the Mental Deficiency Acts of 1913 and 1927). Beginning with the Vagrancy Acts of 1713 and 1744, on the one hand, and with the Madhouses Act of 1774, on the other, two streams of statutes sought to provide means of admitting both pauper and paying patients to institutions and of controlling and improving standards within those institutions. Historians may differ as to the true reasons underlying the asylum movement of the eighteenth and nineteenth centuries,[38] but it is common ground that the prerogative procedures were not used and were not thought suitable to be used for the great majority of patients. Further, although the legislation allowed for the admission of "Chancery lunatics" (as they were commonly but perhaps inaccurately called) to institutions, it also provided a rather more convenient method of admission, and thus removed any need there might otherwise have been to resort to the prerogative for the sole purpose of providing for the care, treatment or detention of the patient.

The Mental Health Acts 1959 and 1983

By the 1950s when the modernisation of all this legislation was under discussion, the jurisdiction to protect the property of the mentally disordered was, of course, still in use, but there were apparently only 16 people who were under the jurisdiction of a committee of the person. Hence the 1959 Act established the jurisdiction and powers of the Court of Protection to deal with the property and affairs of a patient who was adjudged incapable of managing them for himself. There is clearly some overlap between property and personal affairs, for example where the court may direct the use of the patient's assets to maintain him in a particular home or hospital, or where the court may conduct divorce or other proceedings on his behalf. Generally, however, issues relating to the care and treatment of the patient are dealt with under the quite different compulsory procedures for hospital admission or guardianship.

The provisions of the 1959 (and now the 1983) Act dealing with the jurisdiction and powers of the Court of Protection do appear to be a complete code. They no longer refer to or assume the existence of any royal prerogative. All the previous legislation dealing with it, including the relevant parts of "The Statute Praerogativa Regis" (for which no date is given) is repealed.[39] There is no provision (akin to section 104 of the Children Act 1975) expressly preserving it. Such a provision might have proved hard to explain. Stripped of centuries of legislation and case law based on *praerogativa regis*, what exactly were the Crown's powers? They would certainly contrast oddly with the generally liberal tone of the rest of the Act. Neither is there any provision expressly abrogating the prerogative. Most probably it was felt that it would still exist, but that the legislation had covered all the necessary ground. That being so, the Royal Warrant under which the prerogative was delegated was revoked in 1960.

There are at least two reasons why it might appear in 1959 that the Mental Health Act had made any use of the prerogative, even in relation to the person, unnecessary. First, it did indeed look as though the Act had provided comprehensively for all kinds of decisions to be made on behalf of permanently or seriously disordered patients. The definition of mental disorder may have left some gaps, but long term powers could be exercised over the mentally ill and the severely handicapped. Those powers included long term admission to hospital or reception into guardianship. A guardian enjoyed the same powers over the patient as did the father of a child under 14.[40] This would certainly be adequate to provide consent to medical treatment in most cases. Secondly, however, the legislation was strangely silent on the question of consent to treatment. It was probably assumed that compulsorily admitted patients could be treated without consent, at least if they had been admitted "for treatment" under the Act.[41] It was probably also assumed that non-protesting patients could be treated without formality. The whole aim of the Act was to keep formalities to a minimum, as these were regarded as both inconvenient and stigmatising, and to allow the professionals to proceed on the basis of their professional judgment wherever possible.[42] However strange this may seem to rights-minded lawyers, we should not underestimate the strength and persuasiveness of the view that this is indeed a preferable approach.

The amendments made in 1982 and then consolidated in the Mental Health Act 1983 represented something of a return to the rights-based lawyers' approach.[43] They restricted the scope of compulsory powers, they increased the protection involved in the procedures, and they dealt expressly with the question of consent to treatment for those compulsorily admitted to hospital. However, at the same time, they reduced the scope of long term procedures in relation to mentally handicapped people, they reduced the powers of guardians, and they did nothing to deal with the question of consent to treatment for the informal incapable patient. Whereas the 1959 Act would have provided some solution to the problems in *Re B.* and *T* v. *T*, supposing that they had at that stage been perceived, the 1983 Act provided no solution at all.

The Prerogative Dead or Dormant?

It is tempting to argue that, as the 1959 Act appeared to cover all the ground which had been covered by the prerogative, and in a manner which was then thought preferable, the prerogative itself has been abrogated and could not be revived by the modifications in the 1983 Act.

Parliament can no doubt legislate to abolish a prerogative in this way, but did not do so expressly in this case. Alternatively, it may retain the prerogative but regulate how it is to be exercised. The nineteenth and twentieth century legislation referred to earlier[44] regulated the exercise of the prerogative, expanded or clarified the powers available, and conferred analogous powers in relation to wider categories of people. Yet again, Parliament may replace the prerogative with a statutory scheme which supersedes and may therefore curtail or expand it. This would now appear to be the position with respect to the "property and affairs" of a mentally disordered person. Part VII of the 1983 Act has all the appearance of falling within the principle enunciated by Lord Parmoor in *Attorney-General* v. *De Keyser's Royal Hotel*:[45]

> "The constitutional principle is that when the power of the executive to interfere with the property or liberty of subjects has been placed under Parliamentary control, and directly regulated by statute, the executive no longer derives its authority from the Royal Prerogative of the Crown but from Parliament, and that in exercising such authority the executive is bound to observe the restrictions which Parliament has imposed in favour of the subject."

At first sight, that principle appears equally applicable to the Act's scheme of compulsory powers over the person, for these are undoubtedly thought to deal with the "liberty of the subject." There is no longer any suggestion, as there was with the earlier legislation, that they exist alongside an alternative prerogative jurisdiction. When, for example, Parliament carefully prescribed the conditions under which psycho-surgery could be performed, could it seriously be said to have intended to leave open some alternative power to authorise it under the Royal Prerogative?

This line of reasoning seems highly persuasive in relation to particular issues which are dealt with in the Act. Once we turn to matters which quite clearly are *not* dealt with in the Act, we are faced with the problem of deciding whether Parliament intended to limit the executive's powers to what was there or whether it intended to leave open an alternative source of power. The "Catch 22" is obvious. If the statute gives power to do all that the prerogative allows, then the statute may prevail; but if it does not, then the prerogative still survives. However, the "Catch 22" is only so alarming if this is looked upon as a matter of civil rights and the "liberty of the subject." It could be argued that the prerogative was concerned with people who had been found (after inquisition) not to be ordinary subjects, endowed with the usual legal rights and duties, at all. Such an argument, if accepted, could form some theoretical basis for distinguishing these quasi-parental prerogative powers from others. Although their origin, scope and nature were quite different, they have been likened[46] to the court's inherent powers over children. These were described by Lord Eldon in the well-known case of *Wellesley* v. *Duke of Beaufort*[47] as belonging to the Crown as *parens patriae*, and "founded on the obvious necessity that the law should place somewhere the care of individuals who cannot take care of themselves." The case had nothing to do with the prerogative relating to mental disorder, but clearly the rationale for both could be the same,[48] even if the content and machinery were not.

That being so, the courts might well be tempted to apply similar reasoning to the relationship between statute and prerogative. The cases dealing with the relationship between the statutory powers of local authorities and the prerogative jurisdiction over wards of court have reached the following position.[49] The statutory powers of local authorities do not oust the prerogative jurisdiction. Nevertheless, the courts should decline to exercise that jurisdiction in a manner which conflicts with the statutory powers. If, therefore, the local authority objects to the court's intervention in a matter which is within its control, the court should decline to proceed. If, however, the local authority does not object, or actively seeks the court's assistance in the exercise of its powers, or invokes the jurisdiction in order to fill the gaps in its statutory powers, the court may proceed. This reasoning does not permit the court to use the jurisdiction in order to supply any gaps which the statutes have left in the rights of children, parents or relatives. It is entirely possible that a similar position would develop were the prerogative in relation to the mentally disordered to be revived: the jurisdiction might be used to fill the gaps in the statutory powers of the mental health authorities but not to improve the position of the patient or his family under those statutes.

This in itself would give rise to controversy, for the same reasons that the present imbalance in the availability of the wardship jurisdiction has done so. In relation to mentally disordered people, there is perhaps even more reason for concern. The statutory definitions of mental disorder, the procedures to be invoked, and the powers which those procedures allow, have all been quite carefully thought out. The notion that the restrictions could be circumvented, the procedures replaced, and the powers increased because of the revival of an ancient prerogative created for quite different reasons raises serious constitutional issues, quite apart from the more mundane questions which follow.

Resurrection or Revival

The temptation to advise Her Majesty to re-issue the Royal Warrant under the Sign Manual must be considerable, as it would provide a means of solving the particular problems raised in *Re T.*[50] without recourse to legislation. Or would it? At the very least, some answer to the following questions would have to be found.

First, and most important, how is it to be decided who might be subject to the jurisdiction? The argument put forward earlier as to the special nature of *parens patriae* powers could only apply after some proper determination of the subject's status. Would this still not have to be done by the issue of a commission to enquire into the patient's mental condition? It seems unlikely that the Crown could re-assert the power to take away personal status without some decision as to capacity and it could well be argued that the subject has a right at common law to have that issue tried by jury unless there is legislation to modify it. If the Crown could have permitted a single judge of the High Court to determine the issue before, it is difficult to see why all the nineteenth century legislation aimed at simplifying the inquisition procedures was needed.[51]

Secondly, what should be the test to be applied on the enquiry? At common law, the issue was one of idiocy or lunacy, collectively known as being of unsound mind or *non compos mentis.* A certain latitude as to the definition of unsoundness of mind developed during Lord Eldon's time[52] but he also refused to issue commissions of enquiry unless this was for the welfare of the patient.[53] Nineteenth century legislation limited the enquiry to whether or not the subject was at the time of the inquisition of unsound mind and incapable of managing himself or his affairs.[54] Further, although the jurisdiction extended over the person of the subject, as its principal foundation was the protection and preservation of property, there seems to have been some doubt as to whether there could be an inquisition if there was no property to be protected.[55] As with wards of court, this may have been a practical matter, in that the court could not provide for anyone itself. The present criterion for the Court of Protection, that the patient is incapable of managing his property and affairs, can certainly be thought too vague and too broad for such drastic intervention.[56]

Thirdly, to whom should the Royal Warrant to oversee the management of such patients be issued? It is clear that the Lord Chancellor had no special claim to this jurisdiction, as opposed to his functions in relation to the commissioning of an enquiry. If it be accepted that any prerogative jurisdiction cannot be exercised so as to conflict with statutory powers, it would seem appropriate to confine it to matters relating to the person of the subject which are not dealt with elsewhere in the legislation. This would suggest that the judges of the Family Division would be more appropriate than those of Chancery. It would, however, lead to what might be thought an undesirable division of functions between the Chancery Division judges who sit in the Court of Protection and the Family Division judges who might exercise these powers.

Fourthly, once the jurisdiction has been assumed over a particular person, how is it to operate? In the olden days it appears that the assumption of power was total, as indeed it is now in relation to the property and affairs of a patient under the jurisdiction of the Court of Protection. The powers of the committee of the person seem to have encompassed everything to do with the custody, care and treatment of the patient,[57] although the 1890 Act introduced a requirement of regular five yearly medical certificates, without which the commitment of the person (but not the estate) would lapse.[58] The paraphernalia of a committee of the person could be useful in some cases, but in others it could be an unnecessary sledgehammer if all that is required is a solution to a particular problem.[59] Questions of compatibility with the role of other bodies under the mental health legislation would also arise. Should commitment of the person under the prerogative last indefinitely, when other compulsory powers are subject to regular automatic renewal and review?

Fifthly, if the main practical problem which is giving rise to the calls for revival is the reluctance of some doctors to perform abortions or sterilisations upon adult handicapped people, is this the right forum and the right machinery to solve it? Are the courts really capable of assembling for themselves all the facts, opinions and arguments which may be relevant to deciding that issue in any particular case? The reported decisions so far do not suggest that the courts will find this easy unless there is someone to raise objections to the procedure and back it up with evidence and argument. Might it not be suggested that procedures comparable to those established to decide issues of compulsory treatment under the Mental Health Act are at least as likely to lead to a satisfactory result?

Sixthly, even if we can be satisfied on all these points, is it a practical solution to the problem? Can we at one and the same time hold that these decisions can be taken in accordance with "good medical practice" by doctors alone and that the prerogative powers of the Crown should be revived in order to protect those patients who are incapable of protecting themselves against such interferences with their normal legal rights? In this context, is there not some force in the "Templeman doctrine?" He was speaking only of sterilisation, which in terms of ethics and human rights can undoubtedly be distinguished from other forms of medical treatment or interferences with the person. The difficulty is, however, that the English law of battery is the same no matter what form the treatment takes, at least once it goes beyond what is "acceptable in every day life." Will all decisions have to go to the High Court, or at least will the High Court have to be asked to appoint a committee of the person for all patients who are incapable of taking personal decisions for themselves? After all, it is not possible to interfere with the property and affairs of an incapable person without the authority of the Court of Protection or, now, an enduring power of attorney. Yet surely there is reason to believe that parents who wish to receive and spend a legacy for the benefit of a handicapped person are as likely to be acting in that person's best interests as is, say, a dentist who wishes to take all his teeth out? Placing the burden of all this on the courts, let alone the High Court, is obviously not practical.

This is not to suggest that some more commonly employed protective machinery to cater for the needs of severely handicapped adults would not be desirable. I have long argued that it is.[60] There is every reason to believe that at present decisions are taken on their behalf and their ordinary legal rights are understandably interfered with, without any legal warrant or formalities. But we should not forget that all the efforts of the nineteenth century reformers, whatever their motives, were directed towards providing more practical, less stigmatising, more expert but less elaborate methods of providing for the needs of mentally disordered people than the prerogative jurisdiction had been able to supply. With all its faults, cannot the same still be said of the Mental Health Act? Perhaps we should be thinking of building upon that, and experience of guardianship elsewhere, rather than returning to the past.

Notes

* My thanks to Lloyd Tamlyn for all his help in the early stages of preparing this paper. Errors and views are all my own.
1 (1984), pp. 203–4.
2 [1987] 2 W.L.R. 1213, (H.L.).
3 [1988] 2 W.L.R. 189, 204.
4 P.D.G. Skegg, *Law, Ethics and Medicine* (1984), pp. 72–73; *cf. Wilson* v. *Pringle* [1987] 1 Q.B. 237, *per* Croom-Johnson L.J. at p. 252.
5 See ss.2, 3, 1(2) and 63 respectively.
6 See ss.7, 1(2) and 8 respectively.
7 See *e.g. Gillick* v. *West Norfolk and Wisbech Area Health Authority* [1986] A.C. 112, *per* Lord Scarman at p. 181, *per* Lord Templeman at p. 200; *Wilson* v. *Pringle* [1987] 1 Q.B. 237, *per* Croom-Johnson L.J. at p. 252; see also *Marshall* v. *Curry* [1933] 3 D.L.R. 260; *Parmley* v. *Parmley* [1945] 4 D.L.R. 61; *Murray* v. *McMurchy* [1949] 2 D.L.R. 442.
8 [1987] 1 Q.B. 237, at 252 (the case was about horseplay between schoolboys).
9 [1984] 1 W.L.R. 1172, at 1177–1178 (the case was about a police officer detaining a woman without arresting her).
10 May 14, 1987.
11 *The Times*, June 4, 1987.
12 *Mental Health Services, Law and Practice* (1986) para. 20.16.1; see also Skegg, *op. cit.*, p. 105.
12a *Op cit*, note 3, pp. 203–204. At p. 199, he defines this as "a situation where based on good medical practice there are really no two views of what course is for the best."
13 *Imperial Tobacco Ltd.* v. *Attorney General* [1981] A.C. 718, *per* Viscount Dilhorne at p. 741; *per* Lord Lane at p. 752.
14 [1987] 2 W.L.R. 1213, at 1218.
15 United Nations, Declaration on the Rights of Mentally Retarded Persons, General Assembly Resolution 2865 (xxvi) of December 20, 1971, articles 1 and 7.

[16] See N. Lowe and R. White, *Wards of Court* (2nd ed. 1986), paras. 1–13 *et seq.*; Law Commission W.P. No. 101, *Wards of Court* (1987), Part III.

[17] [1970] A.C. 668.

[18] [1976] Fam. 185.

[19] The major sources for this account are H.S. Theobald, *The Law relating to Lunacy* (1924), pp. 1–63 and H.M.R. Pope, *The Law and Practice of Lunacy* (1st ed. 1877 and 2nd ed. 1890); see also Halsbury's *Laws of England*, 4th ed. vol. 8, para. 901; F. Pollock and F.W. Maitland, *The History of English Law* (1968 ed.) vol. 1, p. 481; W. Holdsworth, *A History of English Law*, vol. 1, pp. 473–476; W. Blackstone, *Commentaries on the Laws of England* (11th ed. 1811), pp. 303–305.

[20] See "The 'Praerogativa Regis' " in *The Collected Papers of Frederick William Maitland* (ed. H.A.L. Fisher, 1911) vol. II, pp. 182–189, at 183; one Robert Walrond is thought to have procured the royal assumption of rights in respect of the land of natural fools because he wished to prevent his lands falling into the hands of his feudal lord as would at that stage have happened had his idiot heir been equated with an infant.

[21] The text given here is that cited by Theobald, *op. cit.* at pp. 1–2.

[22] W. Blackstone, *Commentaries on the Laws of England* (11th ed. 1811), pp. 303–305.

[23] (1603) 4 Co.Rep. 123, *per* Coke C.J. at 126.

[24] For the text of the Royal Warrant under the Sign Manual delegating the exercise of the prerogative powers, see Theobald, *op. cit.* p. 14.

[25] s.108 refers to the people "for the time being entrusted by the Sign Manual of Her Majesty with the care and commitment of the custody of the persons and estates of lunatics;" s.12 allows the committee of the person to admit the patient to an institution.

[26] Hence Lord Campbell's view that he could do this part of the operation irrespective of the authority delegated by the Sign Manual, Campbell, *Lives of the Chancellors*, vol. 1, p. 14.

[27] *Op. cit.*, p. 23 *et seq.*

[28] See Lunatic Commissions Act 1833 (3 & 4 Will. 4, c. 36); superseded by the Lunacy Regulation Act 1853 (16 & 17 Vict. c. 70); Lunatics Law Amendment Act 1862 (25 & 26 Vict. c. 111); superseded by the Lunacy Act 1890 (53 & 54 Vict. c. 5), amended by the Lunacy Acts of 1891 (54 & 55 Vict. c. 65), 1908 (8 Edw. 7, c. 47) and 1911 (1 & 2 Geo. 5, c. 40).

[29] *Ridgway* v. *Darwin* (1802) 8 Ves. J. 65; 32 E.R. 275.

[30] *Re Wilson* (1831) 2 Coop. T. Cott. 208; 47 E.R. 1129; see also *Re Astley* (1831) 2 Coop. T. Cott. 207; 47 E.R. 1128; Lord Lyndhurst took the same view, *Ex p. Ridgway* (1828) 5 Russ. 152; 38 E.R. 985.

[31] See *e.g.* Lunacy Act 1890, s.116.

[32] (1873) 9 Ch. Ap. 89, *per* James L.J., at 92.

[33] See *Vane* v. *Vane* (1876) L.R. 2 Ch. 124 where Jessel M.R. asserted the power to appoint a guardian, but did not do so.

[34] Pope, *op. cit.*, p. 218; Theobald, *op. cit.*, p. 275.

[35] [1969] 2 Ch. 1.

[36] Following *Re Grimmett's Trusts* (1887) 56 L.J. Ch. 419 and *Re Taylor* (1861) 2 De G.F. & J. 125; 45 E.R. 570.

[37] [1898] 2 Ch. 378.

[38] *Cf.* K. Jones, *A History of the Mental Health Services* (1972) and A. Scull, *Museums of Madness: The Social Organisation of Insanity in Nineteenth Century England* (1979); see also C. Unsworth, *The Politics of Mental Health Legislation* (1987) esp. Chap. 3.

[39] ss.1 and 149(2) and Sched. 8.

⁴⁰ 1959 Act, ss.4(2), 26, 33 and 34(2).
⁴¹ s.26.
⁴² *Report of the Royal Commission on the Law relating to Mental Illness and Mental Deficiency 1954–1957* (Chairman: Lord Percy), Cmnd. 167 (1957); Jones, *op. cit.*; Unsworth *op. cit.*, Chaps. 8 and 9.
⁴³ Unsworth *op. cit.*, Chap. 10.
⁴⁴ See note 27 above.
⁴⁵ [1920] A.C. 508, at 575; See Heywood & Massey, *Court of Protection Practice*, (11th ed. 1985 by N.A. Whitehorn), at p. 5.
⁴⁶ *E.g.* in Halsbury, *op. cit.*, and in *Re Eve* (1986) 31 D.L.R. (4th ed.) 1, a decision of the Supreme Court of Canada; see also A. Grubb and D. Pearl, "Sterilisation and the Courts" [1987] C.L.J. 439, at 458–464.
⁴⁷ (1827) 1 Russ. 1, at p. 20; 38 E.R. 236, at 243.
⁴⁸ In *Ex p. Cranmer* (1806) 12 Ves. Jun. 445, at p. 449, 33 E.R. 168, at 170, Lord Erskine stated that "the whole prerogative is this, that it falls to "the King to take care of those, who cannot take care of themselves."
⁴⁹ *A.* v. *Liverpool City Council* [1982] A.C. 363; *Re W.* (*A Minor*) (*Wardship: Jurisdiction*) [1985] A.C. 791; see also *Re M.* [1961] Ch. 328.
⁵⁰ [1988] 2 W.L.R. 189; see also Grubb and Pearl, *loc. cit.*
⁵¹ See note 27.
⁵² See *Ridgway* v. *Darwin* (1802) 8 Ves. J. 65; 32 E.R. 275, where Lord Eldon acknowledged that if the issue is not absolute insanity "certainly many difficult and delicate cases with regard to the liberty of the subject occur upon that"; see also *Ex p. Cranmer* (1806) 12 Ves. Jun. 445; 34 E.R. 168; *cf. Ex p. Barnsley* (1744) 3 Atk. 168; 26 E.R. 899.
⁵³ *Ex p. Tomlinson, ex p. Broadhurst* (1812) 1 Ves. & Bea. 57; 35 E.R. 22.
⁵⁴ Lunacy Regulation Act 1862, s.3.
⁵⁵ Theobald *op. cit.*, pp. 19–20; the costs of the inquisition and the later administration came out of the estate.
⁵⁶ L. Gostin, *The Court of Protection* (MIND, 1983).
⁵⁷ Pope *op. cit.*, (1877), Chap. X.
⁵⁸ s.115; Theobald, *op. cit.*, at p. 46 makes the revealing remark that "The section was introduced into the Act of 1889 to meet the anxieties which then existed with regard to the liberty of the subject. It is ill-conceived and causes trouble and expense, it is not wanted and could safely be repealed."
⁵⁹ In a recent Scottish case, the procedure under Scottish common law for appointing a tutor-dative was used to give defined and time-limited powers to the parents of a handicapped adult; see A.D. Ward, "Revival of Tutors-Dative," 1987 S.L.T. 69. Roman law, of course, knew a somewhat similar *curatio furiosi*. Schemes for partial guardianship of mentally handicapped or incapable adults are now being developed in many parts of the world and already exist in Victoria and Alberta.
⁶⁰ *E.g.* "The Rights and Responsibilities of the Mentally Handicapped," (1981) 9 Brit. Inst. Ment. Hand. 67; "The Elderly Mentally Ill and Infirm: Procedures for Civil Commitment and Guardianship", paper at *International Association on Family Law*, 6th World Conference, Tokyo, April 1988.

Ethical Implications of Terminal Care

KENNETH C. CALMAN

Introduction

Ethics is a practical subject, and deals with real problems. It allows clarification of thinking, helps in the analysis problems, and can assist in decision making. The theoretical basis provides the conceptual framework by which ethical dilemmas can be reviewed. Ethical problems in the terminally ill, provide an important example of the kinds of ethical problems which are currently facing doctors and other health care workers. They are concerned not only with the problems of the patient, but those of the relatives, the public at large, and the professionals themselves. In this aspect of medical care, values, beliefs cultural and religious backgrounds are of considerable importance. For a more detailed treatment of some of the issues involved the reader is referred to a burgeoning literature.[1]

In considering the ethical implications associated with the terminally ill it is normal to think of the "big" topics such as euthanasia or suicide. Yet these are not frequent problems faced by the health care team compared with the more common and equally difficult problems of truth telling, quality of life, confidentiality and consent to treatment. This review will therefore deal with a wide range of issues in adults and children with a variety of forms of terminal illness. It begins with an overview of the definitions and concepts which will be used in this chapter.

Basic Concepts and Definitions

The end point of the process of terminal illness is, of course, death. In the group of patients to be discussed in this review, the definition of death does not present the particular kinds of ethical problems associated with organ transplantation and brain death. In all instances the patients have been designated as "terminally ill," and death has been expected, often for a period of time before the event occurs. This does not mean the event itself will occur at a precisely defined time, far from it, rather, that the fact that it might occur in the near future has been considered. This review will not consider further the question of the sudden, unexpected death, in which special methods of diagnosis need to be considered. In general, death in the group of patients under consideration is diagnosed clinically, and without real difficulty.

Far more difficult however, is the definition as to when dying, or the terminal illness begins. It is true of course that the process of dying begins as soon as we are born, but this statement is of little practical value. In general, terminal illness begins when three conditions have been satisfied. First the diagnosis of the illness has been made and other remedial conditions eliminated. Secondly that the advent of death is certain and not too far off. This is a particularly difficult decision to make. Thirdly that medical and nursing effort has turned from the curative to the palliative. This last point is, in effect, the practical way in which the decision that dying is occurring is implemented by the health care team. Each of these three components is fraught with uncertainty, a point which emphasises the distinction between the factual information on which a decision may be based, and which is often incomplete, and the judgement of the professional related to that information. It is the distinction between serious illness, and being seriously ill.

Dying describes the process, or processes, by which death occurs. It has a number of components and a knowledge of these is necessary for a full understanding of the ethical issues involved. These components must be seen in relation to each other and the individual patient viewed as a whole. For example a particular symptom such as pain may be a problem in one patient while in another what would seem to be the same level of pain is less significant because of other features of the illness. Aspects normally included are the physical, emotional, psychological, social, spiritual, and intellectual dimensions of the patient's life. Each of these may be affected in varying degrees during the process of dying. Collectively they form the basis of the quality of life of the individual, a concept of some importance in terminal care.

While the concept of quality of life is a central one it is by no means easy to define. It must relate to individuals, is likely to vary with time, and will depend on past experiences and future expectations. It will be concerned with a whole range of dimensions, not just the physical aspects of the illness. In simple terms quality of life describes the difference between the hopes, dreams and aspirations of an individual, and their present situation. This gap measures the quality of life and is multi-dimensional.[2]

In the field of terminal care the management of uncertainty is a key clinical issue. Thus if we *KNEW* that the treatment would certainly be effective, or that the patient would respond to talking about the issues in a particular way, or that death would occur in eight days precisely, then the task of the doctor would be easy. It is specifically because we do *NOT* know the answers to these, and other similar questions, that the difficulties arise.

Perhaps some examples of the diagnostic difficulties which may occur will illustrate this more effectively. A 55 year old woman with bilateral breast cancer presented with jaundice and pain in the region of her liver. The most likely diagnosis was that the disease had spread to the liver, and that little else could be done for her. However a more careful look at the problem together with some investigations revealed that she had gallstones and required a simple operation to deal with it. A second example was a 60 year old man with stomach cancer, referred for chemotherapy. While on treatment he deteriorated, was unable to eat, and had abdominal pain. Treatment was about to be stopped, but before doing so an x-ray was performed which revealed a non-malignant narrowing of the stomach, the cause of his symptoms. This was corrected by a simple surgical procedure. A third patient was a young woman with breast cancer who developed severe back pain, requiring morphine for control. Investigations showed no obvious cause for the pain and she was put into the category of "advanced disease." However a gynaecologist was asked to see her, and he identified a misplaced intra-uterine contraceptive device which had caused a pelvic infection, resulting in the back pain. A course of antibiotics resolved the pain. These, and many others like them illustrate the concept that "sinister symptons are sometimes simple" and that patients with serious illnesses can develop simple conditions. Even more difficult is the situation of a patient diagnosed as having terminal cancer, who is neither terminally ill nor has cancer.[3]

The other major uncertainty is that of prognosis. Perhaps the commonest question asked by patients or relatives of patients who are terminally ill is "How long have I to go?" This question is almost impossible to answer and is full of uncertainty. Even within hours of death it is possible to be quite wrong[4]. Clearly experience is a help, but even this can be misleading. The fact that it is not possible to answer such a simple question with any degree of certainty is the cause of much misunderstanding between patients and professionals. The question does require an answer, but it is often necessary to be vague and imprecise at best and more usually it is more honest to say "I don't know." Thus, even the most basic components of the definition of terminal illness, the diagnosis and the prognosis, can be subject to uncertainty, making the ethical problems which result, difficult to deal with. For those outside the health care professions this can be difficult to understand, as it is sometimes assumed that the basic information (the facts) is clear and unequivocal, and that indecision is based on a lack of ethical judgement. In practice the opposite can be the case.

The final area to be discussed is the range of conditions which can come within the ambit of "terminal illness." First it should be made clear that all age groups are involved, children, adolescents, adults and the elderly. While there are a number of common problems there are some aspects which are specific to each group. Secondly the term "terminal illness" should be taken to include a wide range of illnesses including cancer, heart and lung disease, Aids and neurological diseases such as stroke or multiple sclerosis. In children there are a specific group of neurological problems, inherited diseases and congenital defects which fit into this category. The term can therefore include any chronic disease associated with a high chance of dying. Thus psoriasis, though a chronic disease, is not normally fatal and would not be included in the definition. Cancer is often taken as the model for "terminal illness" but it should be obvious that this is not the only cause.

The basic concepts of death, dying, quality of life and terminal illness have now been described, and the importance of uncertainty underlined. The next step will be the clarification of the ethical principles involved.

Some Ethical Principles

In the introduction it was noted that an understanding of a broad ethical framework would be of value in the interpreting practical clinical problems. Such issues can be viewed in three ways, each of which is relevant to terminal illness.

(1) The principles are seen in relation to aggregates, populations, communities or special groups. The two major principles here are justice and utility. This is a third person view of medical ethics.
(2) Between individuals such as patients and doctors. Concepts such as compassion, justice and non-maleficence are relevant here. This considers ethical issues in the second person.
(3) Concerned with the morality and integrity of each individual health care professional, the first person view.

Each of these levels is relevant and will be discussed subsequently. Underlining them all, however, is the basic principle of autonomy, a concept which is quite crucial to the understanding of the ethical problems of the terminally ill, including as it does the principles of self determination and self government.

These principles, of course, relate to deeper, and very fundamental problems such as "Why has this happened to me?" or "Why did God let this happen?" Such questions also occur to those caring for dying patients as their own mortality is questioned each time a patient in their care dies. This is a major source of stress in the caring professions. These moral, ethical and spiritual problems must be seen separately from the legal issues which also arise in patients who are terminally ill. While they are clearly connected it is important at certain levels that they are not confused.

In describing the concepts and definitions involved in terminal illness, and the ethical framework in which the clinical problems can be placed, it should be clear that the subject is a complex one, with no simple solutions or easy answers. The next section will deal with some of the commoner ethical problems faced by those caring for the terminally ill. It does so in relation to the three levels of ethical problems described above.

Ethical Aspects of Terminal Care in the Community

This section is concerned mainly with the principles of justice and utility. It is clear in reviewing the services available for the care of the terminally ill, that there are important inequalities in the service in at least two respects. The first is that facilities available are very unequally distributed. In some parts of the country there are a number of hospices, district nursing services and home care teams. In others these are just not available. In many instances it is the charitable organisations who fund this service and the financial input from the Health Authorities limited. The growth of the service often depends on the enthusiasm of individuals or small groups, rather than the needs of the community.

The second reason for the inequality is that while some forms of chronic disease are relatively well served, notably cancer, other forms of illness such as stroke or multiple sclerosis are generally poorly served. It is much easier, for example, to get a night nursing service for a cancer patient, than for an elderly patient with a stroke. The public perception is that cancer patients require care and support and are therefore worth resourcing, while in the public's eyes, other terminal illnesses are less deserving. This has been brought into even sharper focus with the need to develop support services for Aids patients. Whereas communities might be pleased to have within their midst a hospice for cancer patients they seem, on the evidence so far, to be less willing to have one for Aids patients. This poses major ethical questions for the community at large, and not just for the caring professions. How many hospices do we need? Who should be admitted to such places? This is also related to the personal morality of individuals and their integrity. There is some evidence, however, of discrimination in this area.

The second important principle is that of *utility*. This has a particular poignancy in the care of the terminally ill, where the cost of one dying person is counted against the needs of the population as a whole. In a world in which there are diminishing resources for health care with an increasing need to take on new services and developments, it would be surprising if the costs of the care of the terminally ill had not been scrutinised from an utilitarian point of view. How can you justify putting resources into terminal care of the cancer patient and not consider the present inadequacies of the cervical screening programme, or the amount of resources devoted to cessation of cigarette smoking? These are difficult questions to answer and the answer must surely lie some where in the middle. Individuals with some form of terminal illness have a right to expect that care will be provided for them. If it is not, then it is not surprising that individuals in this position may feel that they are a burden on their loved ones, and society as a whole. Public pressures and resource allocation may force patients to consider the costs of their own care to the community.

This comment leads naturally into a discussion of the ethical problems associated with relationships between patients and professionals, and their families.

Relationships in Terminal Care, Ethical Implications

An essential feature of relationships between patients and health care professionals is the consultation. This is the main point of contact between individuals and is the focus of any communication. Communication in this sense is seen as a two-way process during which the skills of the health professional are matched to the needs of the patient. There is time for discussion and to build up mutual trust. This is essential if there is to be any kind of sharing of information and to preserve control by the patient over decision making. In a similar way, many of the inter-professional ethical problems boil down to personal relationships between individuals, and the same principles of building up trust also hold. At a practical level it is difficult to discuss ethical principles without some understanding of inter-personal relationships.

The most important ethical principles in relationships are those of compassion, justice, non-maleficence and autonomy. This latter principle being fundamental to any relationship, and is concerned with the need for individuals to be self determining and self governing. In patients who are terminally ill autonomy is a crucial issue.

Perhaps the commonest problem which faces the doctor or the nurse in relation to autonomy is that of truth telling. On the face of it this would seem to be an uncomplicated issue. The patient is dying, has a right to know the truth, why not tell? In an ideal world this would certainly be the case, but there are a number of uncertainties. What is the truth? Will the patient listen? What effect will it have on the patient? It is questions like these which go through the mind of the doctor. The situation is further complicated by the involvement of the relatives who often ask that the diagnosis is withheld from the patient. In some instances it happens that the relative is told of the diagnosis before the patient. This may occur, for example, on the evening following a surgical operation, while the patient is still under sedation or the effects of the anaesthetic. While the relatives do have a right to be involved, they do not have the right to determine treatment, or what is told to the patient. With these complicating factors, together with the uniqueness of individual patients, how is the doctor to respect the patients' autonomy? Patients do have rights and they have to be respected, but how?

Perhaps the first principle is that patients should not be told lies. Almost all doctors would agree with this. But does this mean that one should always tell the truth? Perhaps not necessarily. On what basis then should the truth be withheld? The principles of compassion and not-maleficence are often invoked at this point to override autonomy. But this is dangerous ground, and can raise the spectre of paternalism. A difficult ethical problem is in respecting the wishes of the relatives. Most doctors faced with this problem, will normally agree to their wishes, but will add the proviso that if the patient asks, the truth will be forthcoming.

If truth has been withheld it can add tension and stress to the caring team. Individual members of the team may be placed in an impossible situation in which they may have to lie to keep up the pretence. In effective teams it would be expected that such problems would be discussed beforehand and an agreement reached.

In some instances the most appropriate response is to admit that the doctor does not know the answer to the question. This is not always easy to do, as it might change the patient-doctor relationship. It does require courage, and a degree of maturity and self-confidence.

So far we have been concerned with the question of truth telling. Another important issue related to autonomy is that of consent to treatment and procedures. In those patients who are terminally ill treatment for curative purposes is not appropriate. However situations may arise when treatment for palliation may be desirable. For example, in a patient with severe bone pain, the most appropriate treatment might be radiotherapy. This in itself is straightforward to administer, but may require the patient to travel, or be admitted to hospital, at some distance from home. Under these circumstances it is obviously essential that the patient is given full information on which to make a decision about treatment. This will also apply to drug treatment. During the last few weeks of life, drugs of various sorts may be considered necessary for the control of symptoms. Informed consent is required. This does imply however that the diagnosis has been discussed, and that the patient is aware that he or she is dying.

Although it is not commonly discussed, there is a great need for research of various kinds in relation to terminal care. We badly need better drugs for the control of symptoms; new methods of controlling psychological distress are urgently required; an investigation of the problems of bereavement might add greatly to our ability to help families; studies of the blood levels of pain killing drugs may assist in making their use more effective. Many other examples could be given, suffice it to say that research is necessary if we are to improve the care of the terminally ill. But is it ethical in the terminally ill? If not, how does this group of patients differ from other groups in which it is legitimate to carry out research? What special precautions would be required? In general it is fair to say that given adequate safeguards of informed consent, it is possible to do research on this group of patients. It is essential however that the implications are fully discussed with the patient, the relatives and the caring team. This latter is essential if there is not to be friction between members of the team. The view of consent expressed here is that of an extension of the doctor-patient relationship, rather than as a legally restrictive device.[5]

This also leads to an examination of the role of the research worker in this situation. Suppose, for example that a nursing research project is set up to observe the time spent by nurses in carrying out a particular task. It becomes obvious that one nurse consistently mishandles the problem. The research worker must either intervene, and thus destroy the research, or leave patients to suffer. The dilemma would normally be resolved by intervening on behalf of the patient. The observer, therefore is very much part of the experiment.

The most widely discussed issue involving autonomy, is euthanasia. At the outset, it is necessary to consider what is meant by the term. Indeed it might even be worth abandoning the term altogether. Literally it means a good death, but over the years the word has gathered overtones which have modified this meaning. It is now associated with an active attempt to end life, normally initiated by the patient. Euthanasia in the original sense would be acceptable to all doctors; a good death, symptom free, and with dignity would be supported by all. This would not be the case with the second definition. The World Medical Association have considered this second sense of the word and issued the statement.

"Euthanasia, that is the act of deliberately ending the life of a patient, either at his own request, or at the request of his close relatives is unethical. This does not prevent the physician from respecting the will of the patient to allow the natural forces of death to follow its course in the terminal phase of sickness."[6]

This statement might not be accepted by all doctors, and the phrase "at the request of his close relatives" is a very controversial one.

This report distinguishes between two types of euthanasia, active and passive. The active one involves a specific action on behalf of the doctor, directed towards ending the life of the patient. The passive one concerns the non-treatment of potentially remediable conditions, such as an infection. In essence this is the distinction between "acts and omissions." An important ethical question is whether or not there is a distinction between these two. Is it morally right to withhold treatment which might result in the death of the patient, while it would be abhorrent to administer a treatment which might end the patients life? Or could both views be considered to be wrong?

Much of this argument centres around the question of quality of life, and the wishes of the patient. The first, as has been stated before, is difficult to define, but must be related to the individual's perception of their life. The second is clearly concerned with the autonomy of the patient. How does the doctor resolve these conflicts, particularly if the patient asks that his life be terminated? Most doctors will act according to their own code of values (emphasising the importance of personal moral values) and take into account the uniqueness of the patient. This does require that there is openness and trust in the relationship. Doctors are not there to play God, rather to serve the patient and the community. In the majority of instances with discussion, and time, a mutually agreed plan can be worked out. The difficulty arises if the patient's wishes are not met by the doctor in the case of euthanasia. From personal experience it is not a common event to be asked to end the life of a patient, though at some time, most doctors have been asked to do this. In the Netherlands there is legislation which allows this to be carried out.

When the symptoms are severe, for example in association with extreme pain, the doctor will normally try to relieve this by using drugs or injections to control the pain. In doing so the life of the patient *may* be shortened, but this can be justified by the doctrine of double effect. This doctrine states that if the primary effect of a treatment is to relieve symptoms then the secondary effects, for example the shortening of life, may be acceptable. This is an uncomfortable doctrine as it points the finger at the side effects of treatment. Most doctors would consider however that this was legitimate in striving for a good death, and in preserving quality of life. There are alternatives to euthanasia which range from taking all possible steps to preserve life, to carrying out an act which

might, as a secondary consequence, shorten life. Doctors are not
in the business of prolonging the act of dying, nor in the act of
deliberate killing. If the patient expresses a wish to commit suicide
the doctor may not facilitate this, as this is a criminal offence.
Therein lies the ethical dilemma. One method which is occasionally invoked is that of the "my mother" principle. This asks the
health care worker to consider the patient as if she were his mother
and to make a decision accordingly. There are naturally inherent
dangers in this approach.

   Associated with the issue of euthanasia is the principle of non-
maleficence, "first do no harm." In the management of patients
with terminal illness treatment and investigations may do harm.
Their purpose, of course is to elucidate the problem, or to treat a
particular sympton. However in doing so the patient may
experience discomfort, either physical or psychological. The
answer here, as in other areas is to have a proper relationship with
the patient in order that the advantages and disadvantages of the
treatment can be fully discussed and a joint decision made. The
partnership aspect of this is important if the autonomy of the
patient is to be respected.

○ A development of importance to the ethical issues associated
with the terminally ill is the concept of the "living will." This is a
document written by the patient while they are well, and outlines
their wishes in the event of serious illness. It adds a new dimension
to moral problems and still requires further discussion.[7] It raises
the question of resuscitation, a topic commonly mentioned by
patients. NTBR (not to be resuscitated) is a wish often expressed
by patients. In those who are terminally ill this may be discussed
with the patient, and in almost all instances would be quite
inappropriate.

   There is debate in the literature as to the importance of ordinary
and extraordinary means in the treatment of the terminally ill.
Extraordinary medical measures have been defined by the Church
Assembly Board (in 1965) as

> "whatever here and now is very costly, or very unusual, or
> very painful or very difficult or very dangerous or if the good
> effects that can be expected from its use are not proportionate
> to the difficulty and inconvenience that are entailed."[8]

   As a general principle this would probably be endorsed by most
doctors. It is in the specifics that it becomes difficult to interpret.
For example does the use of antibiotics, nutritional support,
intravenous fluids or blood transfusion constitute "extraordinary

means" in a group of terminally ill patients? Would a hospice be considered to be an extraordinary means? Many would consider that the use of such methods would be perfectly acceptable to relieve symptoms in some patients. Thus the relief of pleuritic pain from a pneumonia would be more effectively dealt with by an antibiotic rather than morphine. The development of Aids has made this situation even more confused. Such patients may require costly and heroic measures to maintain their quality of life and to allow them to die with dignity. This is a new view of extraordinary means which will challenge our existing assumptions.

Compassion is an important component of the approach of health care professionals to the terminally ill. It has an active element, unlike empathy or sympathy which are more passive. It is concerned with doing the best for the patient. This does, however, raise another issue, which has been discussed before, that of what is best for the patient? Who is to be the judge of that? Again the relationship between the patient and the health care professional is the crucial feature.

Compassion also has another aspect which relates to the personal values of the carer. Involvement in the patient is to be encouraged, but there is a price to pay on behalf of the professional. Stress and "burn out" are common in the group of professionals concerned with the care of the dying[9]. The carers' own lives can become emotionally destroyed by the extent of the involvement with patients. Inter-professional disagreements which might seem trivial can be blown up out of all proportion and the ambience of the clinical unit destroyed. It is not easy to care over a long period of time with this group of patients, particularly if the kind of commitment and compassion which are required for a proper patient-professional relationship are demanded. With this kind of pressure it is not difficult to slip into paternalism and thus avoid the trauma of confronting the patient's autonomy.

The final point to make in relation to patient-professional relationships concerns justice. It is necessary for the doctor or nurse to be aware of the different cultural and religious values of patients, to treat them all with fairness, and to be non-judgemental. Long term cigarette smokers with lung cancer can feel guilty enough without this being reinforced by the doctor. Again the advent of Aids has challenged professionals to look closely at the principle of justice in relation to the deployment of resources, and the nature of the relationship between the patient and the professional. Discrimination is not far from the surface[10].

Personal Ethical Issues

Having discussed the issues which affect populations, and inter-personal relationships, a number of topics which are concerned with the values of the individual health care worker will now be considered. The most obvious is that concerning the doctor's beliefs and values compared to those of the patient. There is scope here for conflict, and one only has to mention Aids, euthanasia and certain religious beliefs to realise that other people's views may be at variance with those of the doctor or the nurse. The important ethical principles here are compassion and justice, and the ability to be non-judgemental, to treat everyone with fairness. This requires a great deal of personal integrity, and a critical self-awareness of one's own views and values. Ethical problems can be very challenging at a personal level, and cause a great deal of heart searching.

Another personal aspect of ethical problems in the terminally ill, concerns disagreements within the team. How does the doctor or nurse deal with views expressed by other health care workers, which differ from their own? Presumably if it is a minor incident, or is a one-off situation, it might be forgotten. But suppose it is not. Suppose it is something about which the individual feels very strongly? Under these circumstances there are several courses to follow, which might include, forgetting about it, confronting the individual, telling the patient or family about the difference of opinion, or even resigning from the post. Some of these require a considerable amount of courage, and could well result in difficult personal career decisions. The phrase of Polonius in Hamlet "to thine own self be true" can be a difficult one to follow.

This last point, however does raise a fundamental issue in dealing with the care of the terminally ill, who should make the choices or decisions?

Whose choice is it anyway?

This is a question which has been widely debated. Two quotations may serve to highlight the problems. The first is from Jonathan Glover in his book *Causing death and saving lives* (1977).

"Only by familiarity with detailed cases, which I lack, is any one likely to work out precise guidelines."[11]

The second is from Ian Kennedy in *The management of terminal illness* (1984).

> "The doctor has no greater expertise than the layman in dealing with ethical issues."[12]

These two statements highlight the dilemma. If the doctor or nurse involved with the patient cannot, or is not competent to make decisions, then who is? First of all let us be clear that it is the patient who has the right to make whatever decisions they wish about their own lives. However it would be naive to think that advice was not sought from those around them, the doctor, the nurse, the minister, the priest, the lawyer, the friend or the family. Who then is competent to make such judgements? Should ethical issues in terminal care be referred to a committee, to a moral philosopher, to society as a whole? In practical terms when patients ask questions or seek advice they want an answer, and, as they often ask the member of the health care team, perhaps it is their responsibility to take part in the process.[13]

A sympathetic view of Kennedy's comment would be that though doctors have no greater expertise than the layman in dealing with ethical issues, they are no worse than the public at large, or indeed in relation to other professional groups. With the increasing teaching of ethics in medical schools it might be anticipated that doctors, and other health care professionals might be better equipped in the future to deal with ethical issues in terminal care as problems certainly exist.[14]

Some special problems

One area of particular concern is the effect that the age of the patient might have on ethical issues, and this would relate especially to the elderly, and to children. Both of these groups may have a particular problem in relation to competence to consent to treatment, procedures, and the ability to fully understand information given to them. In both instances quality of life is a very important issue. It would be fair to say however that both of these groups are very well able to comprehend information, in general, and that we often underestimate their ability to be part of the decision making process.

With dying children, the views of the relatives are of particular concern. The relief of suffering, the preservation of quality of life, may have to be balanced against the possibility of the next new drug miraculously curing the patient. It is often harder to "give up" with children because of the relatives and the attitudes of the caring team.[15] A recent innovation has been the development of hospices for children, and it remains to be seen whether or not this concept will find general acceptance[16].

Children also raise another general problem in the care of the dying, that of the care of patients with non-malignant disease. As was mentioned earlier, the facilities for the care of this group of patients at any age are less well developed than with cancer patients. The reasons for this are unclear. The ethical problems however are the same. Telling the truth, the use of extraordinary means (eg. children with spina bifida), euthanasia (eg. the demented elderly), and consent. Indeed topics such as the policy for resuscitation may be of more relevance in the non-malignant group.

A final general issue is that of confidentiality. This is particularly concerned with the knowledge of the diagnosis, and its dissemination. Cancer, Aids, Multiple Sclerosis etc, are very emotive words, and the privilege of the patient not to have this divulged must be respected. Teams are very valuable, and indeed indispensible in the care of the terminally ill. But how big should the team be? Do all members of the team need to know all the information? The same questions arise with the family and friends. How much information can be released? As before, this is a decision which should be made by the patient, but for many of the practical reasons discussed before the doctor or nurse is often faced with making decisions. Within the team it requires that the level of trust among members of the team is high. Confidentiality may also be of importance at the time of bereavement, when a knowledge of the final diagnosis may be requested by friends, or even the press. With the increase of teaching in terminal illness, confidentiality must be maintained.

Summary and conclusions

This article has reviewed a number of ethical issues relevant to terminal illness. Central to this has been the relationship between the doctor, or other health care worker, and the patient. It is difficult to understand the ethical problems which might arise without an understanding of this relationship. In addition the uncertainty surrounding many of the issues has been highlighted. The questions were raised at three levels, that of the population, at the interpersonal level, and at the level of personal morality. There is a need for greater public debate on the topics raised together with a greater awareness amongst professional groups of the importance of the questions discussed here. For this reason, the greatest need is for broadly based, multi-disciplinary, professional education in philosophy, ethics, logic and law.

In his book "Creative Suffering," Paul Tournier points out that the doctor has two functions.[17] The first is to deal with the immediate situation and relieve the suffering. The second is just as important, however, and that is to help the patient benefit from his illness. Even in those who have a terminal illness there is still the possibility of good quality of life and the hope of being able to achieve personal goals. An understanding of the ethical issues involved can assist in this process.

Notes

[1] R. Gillon, *Philosophical Medical Ethics*, Wiley, 1986; T. Beauchamp and J. Childress, *Principles of Biomedical Ethics*, Oxford U.P., 1979; C. Culver and B. Gert, *Philosophy in Medicine*, Oxford U.P., 1982. See also the new journal, *Bioethics*, 1987.

[2] Calman, K.C., "The quality of life in cancer patients — an hypothesis." (1984) J. Med.Ethics. 10, 124–27.

[3] Rees, W.D., Dover, S.B. and Low-Beer, T.S., " 'Patients with terminal cancer' who have neither cancer nor terminal illness." (1987) 295 *British Medical Journal* 318–319.

[4] Heyse-Moore, L.H. and Johnston-Bell, V.E., (1987) "Can doctors accurately predict the life expectancy of patients with terminal cancer?" *1 Palliative Care* 165–166.

[5] Calman, K.C. and McLean, S.A.M. "Consent, dissent, cement." (1984) 29 Scot. Med. J. 209–211.

[6] World Medical Association, 1987, Lancet (i), 1505.

[7] Higgs, R., "Living wills and treatment refusal" (1987) 295 *British Medical Journal* 1221–2.

[8] Church Assembly Board for Social Responsibility, "Decisions about life and death." (1965) C.A.B.S.R., London.

[9] McCue, J.D., "The effects of stress on physicians and their medical practice." (1982) 306 New Eng. J. Med. 458–463.

[10] Boyd, K. M., "The moral challenge of Aids." (1987) 80 J. Roy. Soc. Med. 281–283; Smith, T., "Aids: A doctor's duty" (1987) 294 *British Medical Journal* 6; Steinbrook, R., Lo, B., Tirpack, J., Dilley, J.W. and Volberding, P.A., "Ethical dilemmas in caring for patients with the acquired immunodeficiency syndrome." (1985) 103 Ann. Int. Med. 787–90.

[11] Glover, J. *Causing death and saving lives*. (1977) (Penguin).

[12] Kennedy, I. McC., "The law relating to the treatment of the terminally ill." In

Saunders, C. (ed.) *The management of terminal malignant disease*. (1984) (Edward Arnold).

[13] C. Faulder, *Whose Body Is it Anyway?* Virago Press, 1984

[14] Ahmedzai, S., "Dying in hospital; The resident's viewpoint." (1982) *British Medical Journal* 285 at 712–714; Calman, K.C. and Downie, R.S. "Practical problems in the teaching of medical ethics." (1987) 13 J. Med. Ethics. 153–156; De Saintonge, D.M.C., Littlejohns, D.W. and Vere, D.W. "Teaching and learning about terminal care." (1986) 20 Med. Education 335–341; Finlay, I.G., (1986). "House officers attitudes towards terminal care." 20 Med. Education. 507–11.

[15] Kohler, J. A. and Radford, M., "Terminal care for children dying of cancer: Quantity and quality of life" (1985) *British Medical Journal* 115–116.

[16] Burne, S.R., Dominica, F. and Baum, J.D. "Helen House — A hospice for children: Analysis of the first year. (1984) 289, *British Medical Journal* 1665–1668.

[17] Tournier, P. *Creative suffering*. (1981) SCM Press.

Conceiving—A New Cause of Action?

ANDREW GRUBB*

A. *Introduction*

Most actions for damages consist of claims for personal injuries or property damage suffered by the plaintiff. The loss of a person has never been the proper subject matter of compensation.[1] Parliament had to intervene in the Fatal Accidents Acts in order to provide some remedy for the loss of a breadwinner.[2]

It might be seen as a matter of some curiosity, therefore, that in the 1980's there has emerged an increasing number of claims brought by parents against the medical profession for the birth of a child. While death is not actionable the courts have accepted, what might be seen as the converse, namely that the "blessed" birth of a child may be. In modern times, we have witnessed an apparent contradiction in a society. Considerable scientific effort is made to improve infertility treatment for those unable to bear children. Yet, those who are able to have children may seek damages for the "blessing" they desire and which, in some cases, they will go to great lengths and personal sacrifice (often financial) to achieve.

The natural desire to found a family may be very strongly felt and yet, also, it is easy to understand that family planning can play a significant part in a couple's financial planning. When that plan goes amiss, the financial consequences can be as catastrophic as the loss of a job. The financial burden of the "unplanned child" can be as worrying and disruptive to the family as would be the lack of children. It should be no surprise that attempts have been made to use the law to redress the balance and claim compensation for the costs and financial burdens of unplanned parenthood.

* I am grateful to Professor Ian Kennedy of King's College, London for his invaluable comments on an earlier draft. I am also grateful to Mr Robert Francis for bringing to my attention many of the relevant unreported cases.

As one might expect, like Coca-Cola and bubblegum, the major producer and exporter of these actions has been the United States.[3] But like most North American phenomenon, it has not taken long for an Atlantic crossing.

Three types of action have emerged. First, the action for "wrongful life" brought by a handicapped child itself. Secondly, there is the associated "wrongful birth" claim of the parents. Both these claims usually arise out of the birth of a handicapped child. The third, and last, type of action is one for "wrongful conception" or sometimes in America called "wrongful pregnancy" which is an action brought by the parents, usually for the conception and birth of a healthy but unplanned child. Legal ingenuity has been stretched to the full in constructing these new causes of action.

B. *The Causes of Action*

1. *Wrongful Life*[4]

A "wrongful life" claim is an action brought by a handicapped child alleging that he should never have been born. The essence of these actions is that the doctor negligently deprived the mother of the opportunity of an abortion so that a child has to live a life of suffering. Its life is literally said to be "wrongful." In the United States these claims were originally rejected,[5] but a number of jurisdictions including California,[6] New Jersey,[7] and Washington State[8] have gone some way in accepting them to the extent that the extra cost of maintaining the child because of its handicap may be claimed even though damages to compensate mere existence (including pain and suffering) are not recoverable.

In England, the Court of Appeal in *McKay* v. *Essex A.H.A.*,[9] rejected such an action at common law. The plaintiff child was born severely disabled because the mother contracted German measles during her pregnancy. There was no suggestion that the doctor employed by the defendants had caused the rubella and hence the child's injuries. Instead, it was argued that the tests carried out on the mother to detect rubella had been negligently performed. As a result it had not been known that the child might be handicapped and so the mother had been deprived of the opportunity to have an abortion.

The Court of Appeal produced an impressive set of cumulative reasons for striking out the plaintiff's claim:[10] first, that the child has suffered no injury because some life is better than none; secondly, that such an action is contrary to public policy because it would undermine the principle of the sanctity of human life; thirdly, that the existence of such actions might encourage abortions and even (arguably) put a doctor under a duty to carry out an abortion and, finally, that the court could not calculate the damages that it would have to award by comparing the child's non-existence (which should have happened) and its present handicapped existence (which actually happened).[11]

In any event, in the Congenital Disabilities (Civil Liability) Act 1976 Parliament has concluded the matter against such actions for births after July 1975[12] unless the negligence occurred, not during the mother's pregnancy, but before conception and impaired either parent in their ability to have a normal healthy child.[13] A modern day example of this would be if the mother were negligently to be given blood containing the AIDS virus prior to becoming pregnant and the foetus (and subsequently the child) were to be afflicted by this terrible disease.[14]

2. *Wrongful Birth*

Usually when a handicapped child has been born because of the alleged negligence of a doctor, the actions have not been brought by the child. Instead, the parents have sued claiming the pain and suffering, the physical injuries and the financial losses suffered as a result of the birth of the child. These actions for "wrongful birth" can be seen as the parental equivalent of the child's "wrongful life" action. The doctor may have failed to prevent the *birth* of the child, perhaps, because he negligently performed an abortion. These were the facts of probably the first English case of this type, *Scuriaga* v. *Powell*[15] in 1979 where the court awarded the mother damages for her pain and suffering, loss of earnings, her capacity to earn and for the impairment of her marriage prospects as a single parent. It is worth noting that she did not claim the costs of rearing the child. An additional claim was brought in *McKay* by the parents of the child for the negligent failure by the doctor to advise that her foetus might be severely damaged because of the rubella contracted by the mother during pregnancy.

These claims have fared better in the English courts. Although the Court of Appeal struck out the child's action, it left the parents' claim intact to be determined on its merits at trial.[16]

3. *Wrongful Conception*

(a) *The Background*

The most common action in this area arises out of the birth of a
healthy child as a consequence of a failed sterilisation operation or
other failed contraceptive measure.[17] In these "wrongful conception" actions, the claim is brought by the parents alleging that the
doctor negligently allowed them to conceive a child. As a
consequence of this, physical injury was caused to the mother
during pregnancy and at birth, which caused financial loss to the
parents in raising the child. When the action concerns a failed
sterilisation operation, the action is one for physical injury with
consequential financial loss to the parent undergoing the
procedure.[18] When the action arises from a failed female operation, it will not be possible to point to any physical injury to the
man and the action begins to take on the mantle of a claim for pure
financial loss.[19]

Quite contrary to the title of this paper, "wrongful conception"
cases are not, in fact, new at all. It is possible to find actions of this
sort going back as far as 1961. In *Waters v. Park*,[20] the plaintiff
underwent a hysterotomy and sterilisation. The sterilisation failed.
Havers J.[21] held that the defendant had not been negligent in
failing to advise the plaintiff of this risk because he had complied
with a competent body of professional practice. This first case was
not a very auspicious start for the "wrongful conception" action
but, as we shall see, on the Court of Appeal's present view of the
law, he got it right.

Similarly, in *Williams v. St. Helens and District H.M.C.*[22] in
1977, a woman who underwent a tubal ligation operation as a
contraceptive measure to sterilise her, claimed that if she had been
warned of the failure rate of such operations she would have taken
other contraceptive measures and avoided pregnancy. Her action
failed because Crichton J., like Havers J. before him, held that the
doctor's failure to disclose was not negligent—an issue we shall
have to return to in some detail later.

However, it was not until the 1980's that "wrongful conception"
actions became more common. The reported cases have increased
where vasectomies performed on men[23] or sterilisation procedures
(such as tubal ligations) performed on women,[24] have gone
wrong.[25]

(b) *Public Policy and Damages*

It should be remembered that in these actions the child is born
healthy. Is it not somewhat perverse that the birth of a healthy

child should be compensated in damages? In the recent case of *Gold* v. *Haringay H.A.*,[26] Lloyd L.J. seemed a little concerned at the state of the law if it allowed such actions[27] and he cited the earlier remarks in *Jones v. Berkshire A.H.A.*[28] in 1986 where Ognall J. said:

> "I pause to observe that, speaking purely personally, it remains a matter of surprise to me that the law acknowledges an entitlement in a mother to claim damages for the blessing of a healthy child. Certain it is that those who are afflicted with a handicapped child or who long desperately to have a child at all and are denied that good fortune would regard an award for this sort of contingency with a measure of astonishment. But there it is: that is the law."

One of the most contentious problems faced by the courts in America and England has been whether public policy prevents the recovery of damages for the upkeep of a healthy child.[29] If the parents' claim was restricted to damages for pain and suffering, injury and directly related costs but did not extend to future support, "wrongful conception" claims would probably not be cost effective since most actions would involve claims for relatively small sums.[30] On the other hand, if upkeep costs are recoverable, the size of awards would be such that the claims would be worth pursuing, especially if the courts are prepared to take realistic figures for the cost of keeping, for example, a teenager and not restrict the quantum of damages to something near social security levels.[31]

The first English case to consider this point directly was *Udale v. Bloomsbury A.H.A.*[32] Jupp J. identified a number of considerations which drove him to the conclusion that it was contrary to public policy to award upkeep costs and so make the doctor the financial father of the child. Many of them he derived from the *McKay* case[33] but he added one or two himself: for instance, that it would be highly undesirable for a child to grow up and learn that a court had declared his or her life to be a mistake, that any award of damages would be offset[34] (and sometimes be extinguished) by a figure to represent the joy of having a child[35]—this would put a premium on "unnatural rejection of womanhood and motherhood" and that the birth of a healthy baby was a time for rejoicing and not litigating.[36]

These views were to have a short-lived influence on the law. Just over a year later in 1984 in *Thake v. Maurice*,[37] Peter Pain J. allowed a couple who brought a "wrongful conception" claim to recover the upkeep costs of their unplanned child. He refused to ride the "unruly horse" of public policy which Jupp J. had jumped astride in *Udale*.

Later in 1984, the Court of Appeal in *Emeh* v. *Kensington and Chelsea A.H.A.*[38] resolved the issue in favour of allowing parents to claim these damages by approving the reasoning of Peter Pain J. in *Thake*. Only the House of Lords can now reverse the trend.[39] Waller L.J. said that "the court should not be too ready to lay down lines of public policy."[40] Purchas L.J. also distanced himself from the *Udale* view,[41]

> "I see no reason for the courts to introduce into the perfectly ordinary, straightforward rules of recovery of damages . . . some qualification to reflect special social positions."

Then, as if to leave us thinking he might believe such qualifications would be appropriate, he passed the buck.[42]

> "If something has to be done in that respect . . . then that is a matter which falls more properly within the purview of Parliament."

As *Emeh* illustrates, the judges are able to point to counter arguments for every pro-public policy argument that is raised. Perhaps, the arguments are too well balanced. There is no clear consensus on what the law ought to allow. In these circumstances, it seems to me that he who bears the burden of proof fails to prove his case. Since it must be those who seek to deny the recovery of upkeep costs who must assert a clear public policy, it must be they who fail to prove their case.

However, in my view the *Thake* and *Emeh* approach to damages may have had a deleterious effect on the development of the law. It may well be that the courts' unease with this position has resulted in the restriction of "wrongful conception'" claims. In several cases, the Court of Appeal has taken a narrow view of the law, making it more difficult for a plaintiff to establish a cause of action whether in contract or negligence. Could this be because the court knows that if the plaintiff succeeds his damages claim (at least for the present) will be unacceptably wide. But is this not a case of the "tail wagging the dog?"

C. *Factual Settings for Wrongful Conception Claims*

A "wrongful conception" action may arise in four factual settings.[43]

1. *Pre-Operative Counselling*

The early cases of *Waters*[44] and *Williams*[45] illustrate the situation where the doctor is negligent in his pre-operative counselling of the patient. This setting has generated the greatest number of cases both in England and abroad. But it is here that patients have been least successful in sustaining their causes of action. It is the difficulties of proving negligence in counsellng that we shall return to later in this paper.

(a) *Inherent Risks*
The doctor may negligently fail to inform the patient of some information which is significant to his or her decision to consent to the sterilisation operation. This may arise from his failure to warn the patient of a natural reversal rate of the operative procedure being undertaken. So, for example, it was alleged (unsuccessfully) in *Gold* v. *Haringay H.A.* that it was negligent not to inform a woman patient that a *post partum* sterilisation operation had a failure rate of between two and six in every thousand. Similarly, in *Thake* v. *Maurice* the claim concerned the risk of failure of a vasectomy operation, although unusually here, the non-disclosure was held to be negligent.

(b) *Alternatives*
On the other hand, the negligence might consist of the failure to advise a patient that alternative contraceptive procedures exist which are less likely to fail. So, it was alleged that the doctor was negligent in *Gold* not to advise the woman patient that her husband could undergo a vasectomy which had a lower failure rate than the sterilisation operation performed on her. In *Palmer* v. *Eadie*[46] it was unsuccessfully argued that a doctor had negligently failed to advise a male vasectomy patient that some methods of carrying out the procedure were more sure to leave him sterile than others. Similarly, in the Canadian case of *Dendaas* v. *Yackel*[47] in 1980, the negligence consisted of a failure to inform a woman patient that there was a procedure that she could undergo which had a lower failure rate.[48]

(c) *Precautions*
The final situation of negligence at the pre-operative counselling stage arose in *Venner* v. *North East Essex A.H.A.*[49] One of the allegations of negligence in this case was that the doctor had failed to advise a woman patient who had ceased to take the contraceptive pill prior to undergoing a surgical sterilisation operation that

she or her husband should, in the meantime, take alternative contraceptive measures. On the facts Tucker J. held that the doctor had warned the patient. In any event there should, arguably, rarely be a need for a warning in this situation since it should be obvious to all but the most obtuse patient that alternative contraceptive measures are needed if pregnancy is to be avoided.[50]

2. *Failure of the Contraceptive Measure Itself*

Sometimes the doctor may negligently perform the sterilisation operation itself. In the cases of *Emeh* and *Udale* the defendants admitted their negligence.[51] Without this admission, a plaintiff would be thrown back to having to prove that the doctor failed to come up to the standards of the "reasonable doctor" exercising the doctor's speciality. This is, of course, the well-known *"Bolam* test."[52] But since "[a doctor] is not guilty of negligence if he has acted in accordance with a practice accepted as proper by a responsible body of medical men skilled in that particular art . . . [and he is not negligent] merely because there is a body of opinion who would take a contrary view,"[53] a plaintiff in cases involving an element of clinical judgment will often have considerable difficulty in proving his case.[54]

A different, but related, factual situation arose in the case of *Troppi* v. *Scarff*[55] in 1971 where the Michigan Court of Appeal upheld a finding that a pharmacist was negligent when he used tranquilisers to fill the plaintiff's prescription for birth control pills with the inevitable result that the plaintiff became pregnant.

3. *Post-Operative Testing*

In the case of male vasectomy operations, the procedure is not immediately effective since there remains a residue of sperm in the body for some period after the operation. It is routine medical practice to carry out sperm tests on samples of semen over a period of time after the operation to ensure sterility. Similarly, in the case of a female operation, it may be negligent[56] not to test any tissue removed to ensure that it actually came from the patient's fallopian tubes. Therefore, a doctor might be negligent in not carrying out these tests or, alternatively, he may negligently perform them. In the United States these two ways of putting the doctor's negligence have been pleaded in a number of cases.[57] In England they formed part of the allegations of negligence in *Pattinson* v. *Hobbs*[58] decided by the Court of Appeal in 1985 on a limitation point.

4. *Post-Operative Counselling*

Not only can a failure to counsel before an operation give rise to liability. A failure to counsel after the operation may also do so. For example, this might arise where the doctor fails to warn a male patient of the need to take alternative contraceptive measures until the post-operative sperm tests prove negative.[59] Possibly, this situation might also arise if a doctor failed to advise a patient that the sperm tests had not proved negative and so, leading the patient to believe he is sterile and the patient fails to continue to take alternative contraceptive precautions.

D. *Liability for Failing to Disclose Risks and Alternatives*

As I observed earlier it is the area of failure to disclose the reversal rate of a proposed sterilisation operation or the existence of an alternative procedure with a lower rate of failure that has generated the most cases.

Three problems confront a patient who wishes to succeed in this type of "wrongful conception" action. First, he must prove that the doctor did not give him a warning and/or did not counsel him on the alternative procedure. Secondly, even if he succeeds in doing this, he must establish that the doctor's failure was negligent or amounted to a breach of contract. Thirdly, the plaintiff must establish that the defendant's negligence caused the damage suffered.

1. *Proof*

It can be different for a patient to prove that no warning was given. The events will have taken place probably many years before the court case. The patient will always face the difficulty, that the courts may be sceptical of his self-serving evidence in court.

This, of course, could equally be true of the doctor. But the doctor will often be in an even worse position. He is very unlikely to remember anything specifically about his consultations with the patient. Ognall J. highlighted the difficulties in these situations in *Jones* v. *Berkshire A.H.A.*[60] when he stated

"To [the doctors] [the plaintiff] was one of hundreds, if not thousands, of patients, and therefore there could in common sense be no possibility of their bringing to mind the actual meetings, still less the full gist of what passed between any one of them and the plaintiff. But to the plaintiff on the other hand this was a matter of especial importance and . . . of unique significance to any caring woman with maternal instincts who is going to be rendered . . . infertile . . . In other words, in a phrase, the plaintiff, in my judgement, is a good deal more likely to remember with clarity that which passed on this special occasion in her life than any one of the professional men who attended her."

As a consequence, Ognall J. preferred the plaintiff's evidence and found that no warning of the risk of reversal of the operation had been given.

(a) *Usual Practice*

Because of the doctor's lack of recollection, he is likely to rely upon his standard practice at the time and argue that because he usually gave a warning, he would have done in the case of this patient. In many of the "wrongful conception" cases doctors have put their case in this way. However, it should not be thought that their evidence of their usual practice will always win the day. In *Thake* v. *Maurice*,[61] the defendant alleged that he had given his usual warning. Peter Pain J. found that he had not, but then, in the absence of any other professional evidence, held that it must be negligent for the defendant not to disclose a risk which he himself thought it proper to inform the patient of but which, in this instance, he had failed to do. The doctor, in other words, by trying to prove his case on the facts, admitted his own negligence.

(b) *Consent Forms*

A further way in which a doctor might seek to prove that he had warned the patient of the risk of reversal, would be by relying on the consent form signed by the patient and usually (though not as a legal necessity), the spouse of the patient. The consent form may serve two purposes.

First, it may contain an express warning of the risk of failure. For example, in *Eyre* v. *Measday*,[62] the plaintiff signed a form prior to her undergoing a sterilisation operation which stated, *inter alia*, that although

"[the operation] is nearly 100 per cent. successful, I appreciate that this cannot be guaranteed . . . "

Could it be said that this was a clear warning? At best, perhaps, it removes any argument that the doctor is guaranteeing the patient's sterility.[63]

Secondly, the consent form may contain a statement that the doctor has given a warning to the patient. While it must always be remembered that, as Bristow J. stated in *Chatterton* v. *Gerson*,[64]

> " . . . it would be no defence . . . if no explanation had in fact been given. The consent would have been expressed in form only, not in reality."

This may be some evidence that a warning was given. One of the standard consent forms now in use includes a provision that the doctor had explained the procedure "including the small risk of pregnancy from a failure of this procedure."

In *Jones* v. *Berkshire A.H.A.* Ognall J. thought this was worthless because it was only signed by the doctor and not by the patient. This is something which, it seems according to Ognall J., may be remedied in the near future. But, what is the difficulty? If the form is only evidence of what was said by the doctor, it is surely not crucial that the patient should sign an acknowledgement—that would obviously be more conclusive and, perhaps, would be essential if the patient was alleged to be *volenti* to the risk?

2. *Establishing Liability*

(a) *Contract*

Because sterilisation operations are often carried out privately, there will often exist a contract between the patient and the doctor. As a result, in addition to a negligence action, a doctor may be sued for breach of contract for failing to disclose a risk of reversal.[65] This is unlike the situation under the National Health Service, where the patient's only remedy would be in the tort of negligence, since there is no contract between an N.H.S. doctor and his patient.[66]

In two cases, *Thake* v. *Maurice*[67] and *Eyre* v. *Measday*[68] the Court of Appeal rejected the argument that a failure to disclose a risk of reversal, together with a statement by the doctors concerned that a vasectomy (in *Thake*) and a female sterilisation operation (in *Eyre*) were "irreversible," amounted to an express or implied contractual guarantee that the doctor would render the patient sterile.[69] The courts construed the word "irreversible" to mean "surgically irreversible" only.[70] No reasonable person would interpret the circumstances as amounting to such a guarantee of sterility.[71] In *Thake* Nourse L.J. said[72]

> "...a doctor cannot be objectively regarded as guaranteeing the success of any operation or treatment unless he says as much in clear and unequivocal terms."

The Court of Appeal reached this conclusion not least because of the impossibility a doctor would have in achieving such a guarantee, having regard to the inexactitudes of medical science.[73] Instead the court held that a doctor's contractual obligation would ordinarily be the same as his tortious duty, namely, a duty to exercise reasonable skill and care. These decisions have the attraction of producing symmetry between National Health Service and private patients seeking sterilisation.

(b) *Misrepresentation*

Flowing on from this, the argument has been rejected that to use the word "irreversible," when the contraceptive procedure is not, is to misrepresent to the patient the effect of the procedure. In *Gold*, the trial judge (Schiemann J.)[74] had held that the "defendants negligently misrepresented to the plaintiff that the operation would render her permanently sterile."[75] The Court of Appeal gave this short shrift. Lloyd L.J. held that this could only be sustained if the court inferred it from the doctor's description of the operation as "irreversible." But this was quite impossible in the light of the decision in *Eyre* v. *Measday*.

Adopting a similar approach, Garland J. in *Worster* v. *City and Hackney A.H.A.*[76] refused to construe the words of a consent form which stated "...we understand that this [the operation] means we can have no more children," as amounting to a misrepresentation of sterility. Instead, the judge said

> "It is essentially a consent to an operation intended to produce sterilisation with an acknowledgement that the intended effect was that the plaintiff... could not have any more children."

In the absence of a clear lie or, exceptionally, a guarantee of sterility (which is unattainable), the law of misrepresentation seems to hold little hope for the plaintiffs in this sort of case.

(c) *Liability in Negligence*

So we must turn back to the question of whether it is negligent to fail to disclose (1) the risks of reversal and (2) the existence of an alternative procedure and its failure rate? In jurisdictions where the courts have held that a doctor must disclose the risks which a "prudent patient" in the plaintiff's position would wish to know, the courts have found non-disclosure in these circumstances to be negligent.

In the American case of *Sard* v. *Hardy*[77] it was held negligent not to disclose to a woman patient that a tubal ligation operation might fail. Similarly, in the Canadian case of *Dendaas* v. *Yackel*[78] it was negligent not to tell the patient that there was another more effective procedure to achieve sterility which might prevent her becoming pregnant.

In England, the House of Lords in *Sidaway* v. *Governors of Bethlem Royal Hospital*[79] held that a doctor's duty of disclosure of risks inherent in a medical procedure is usually the same as his duty in relation to treatment or diagnosis. As we have seen, for treatment and diagnosis cases, a doctor is required to exercise the "reasonable skill and care of the ordinarily competent medical practitioner"—the *"Bolam* test." A doctor will comply with this duty if he acts in accordance with a "competent body of medical opinion" even if there is an equally competent body that disagrees.[80]

However, a majority of the House of Lords in *Sidaway*[81] did not simply accept that medical evidence could determine the scope of a doctor's duty to advise his patients in all cases. The stranglehold of the "professional opinion" has been broken. Lord Templeman, although he did not cite *Bolam*, clearly rejected it since he said[82] "I do not subscribe ... to the theory that the doctor is entitled to decide everything" which, of course, is at the heart of *Bolam*. Lord Templeman thought that, instead, the doctor must provide the patient with sufficient information to enable the patient to make a "balanced judgment."[83]

Lord Bridge (with whom Lord Keith agreed) did not accept that the scope of a doctor's duty of disclosure could be determined solely on the basis of the *Bolam* test in medical advice cases. *Bolam* was applicable to an extent, but in a watered down version in contrast to cases of treatment or diagnosis. The scope of a doctor's duty of disclosure was only to be decided *"primarily* on the basis of expert medical evidence, applying the *Bolam* test."[84] Lord Bridge concluded that in some circumstances a non-disclosure in compliance with professional practice might result in a patient lacking information which was "so obviously necessary to an informed choice" so that, in the absence of a "cogent clinical reason," it would be negligent to fail to make disclosure.[85]

In both *Jones* v. *Berkshire A.H.A.* and *Thake* v. *Maurice*, doctors were found negligent in not disclosing the risk of reversal in female, and male, sterilisation operations respectively. But let us not get carried away by this. In *Jones,* the duty to disclose was admitted by the defendants.[86] In *Thake*, as we have seen, the defendant in effect admitted his own negligence since he had not complied with his own practice of disclosure, and there was no counterbalancing expert evidence to show that some other medical practitioners did not disclose.[87] A claim of negligence was originally pleaded in *Eyre* v. *Measday* but it was not pursued before the trial judge.

In the case of *F* v. *R*,[88] the Supreme Court of South Australia decided that a doctor had not been negligent in failing to disclose to a woman a failure rate of between five in a 1000 and one in a 100. The doctor had complied with professional practice in not disclosing the risk when performing the only medically suitable procedure. King C.J. said[89]

> "...I am of the opinion that the better practice, and that which accords best with the rights and interests of the patient, is that adopted by the doctors who do warn of the possibility, however slight, of subsequent pregnancy. But that is not to say that in following the non-disclosure practice, the [doctor] was in breach of her duty of care to the patient."

Since it will not be difficult for a doctor to call evidence of "a responsible body of medical opinion" which would favour non-disclosure in these cases, the patient must persuade the court to depart from the "exclusive reliance" on professional opinion in the context of sterilisation procedures.

(i) *Asking Questions*

The first, and more limited, instance of this concerns a doctor's duty to *answer questions*.[90] If a patient asks about the risk of failure of a sterilisation or the available alternatives, is he or she entitled to know? After *Sidaway*, it seemed clear that a doctor's duty was more onerous if the patient asked him questions. Subject to the doctor having a "therapeutic privilege" to withhold information dangerous to the patient's health,[91] the doctor would have to "answer both truthfully and as fully as the questioner requires."[92]

However, the Court of Appeal in *Blyth* v. *Bloomsbury H.A.*[93] has put the law in some confusion. The case concerned a patient who had received an injection of the long-lasting contraceptive drug, Depo Provera. She suffered some rather unpleasant side-effects. She complained that she had not been told of these by the doctor when she had specifically asked about side-effects. The trial judge, applying the dicta in *Sidaway*, found for the plaintiff.[94] The Court of Appeal reversed the decision. The Court simply stated that the House of Lords could not have meant to depart from the "*Bolam* test"even in cases concerning specific questioning by the patient. The court held that a doctor did not have to tell a patient everything he knew. In the words of Kerr L.J.

"[an] answer must depend upon the circumstances, the nature of the inquiry, the nature of the information which is available, its reliability, relevance, the condition of the patient, and so forth. Any medical evidence directed to what would be the proper answer in the light of responsible medical opinion and practice—that is to say, the Bolam test—must equally be placed in the balance."

The Court of Appeal has taken a significant step back from the dicta of the Law Lords in *Sidaway*. Perhaps, *Blyth* does not purport to give expert evidence the determinative effect it has elsewhere in medical cases, but a future court is quite likely to interpret it in this way. One thing is sure, the Court of Appeal seemed to confuse the issue of what medical information is available (a technical question for expert evidence), with what answer should be given in the light of that information (a legal normative question for the judge).[95] Graciously, the Law Reporters seem to have confined *Blyth* to the obscurity of the vast volume of unreported cases.

(ii) *Gold v. Haringay H.A.*

A more direct attack on the reliance on expert evidence was made in *Gold* v. *Haringay H.A.*[96]

At first instance,[97] Schiemann J. held that the doctor was negligent when he had not disclosed the risk of failure of a tubal ligation procedure and, further, when he had not advised the patient of the alternative vasectomy procedure (for her husband) which had a smaller risk of failure. First, his Lordship determined that no body of medical opinion would have failed to disclose this information. Secondly, in any event, Schiemann J. held that it was unreasonable to fail to disclose the information even if non-disclosure was approved by some practitioners.

The judge interpreted *Sidaway* as deciding that compliance with an approved professional practice would not be negligent[98] but he went on to distinguish the case as being concerned with *therapeutic* procedures whilst sterilisation operations were *non-therapeutic* in nature. His Lordship took the view that while professional practice would be relevant, it would not be deter-minative because none of the reasons for adopting the doctor-orientated test in *Sidaway* applied in this context. So, he concluded that[99]

> "...the hospital doctors faced with Mrs Gold, a perfectly normal sensible woman with no particular psychiatric social or medical problems, were under a duty [to disclose the information]. I can think of no reason why she should not have had these things mentioned to her..."

The judge's view is a bold one, distinguishing as it does, the leading House of Lords' decision in *Sidaway*.

On appeal, the Court of Appeal undid all Schiemann J.'s good work. First, on the facts the court determined that he had misunderstood the evidence; there *was* a competent body of professional practice which would not have disclosed the information. Secondly, applying *Sidaway*, the court held this was determinative of the issue of breach of duty. The doctors could not have been negligent if they complied with it. It is necessary to take a close look at the reasoning of Lloyd L.J.

The "Bolam Test"

The Court of Appeal criticised the judge for not applying the "*Bolam* test." Lloyd L.J. considered the "*Bolam* test" to be of general application to all professionals and, further, that it applied to all aspects of their professional practice. But, this is an unfair criticism of the judge and it is a misunderstanding of *Bolam*.

The "reasonable professional" test is universal[1] but *Bolam* as interpreted by the House of Lords in the trilogy of cases of *Whitehouse* v. *Jordan*,[2] *Maynard* v. *West Midland R.H.A.*[3] and *Sidaway* itself, as resulted in its being applied in a very different way in medical cases. Normally, compliance with an accepted professional practice is only *some* evidence in favour of the defendant; it is not usually regarded as determinative of the absence of negligence, whether in cases of professional negligence by, for example, bankers[4] or lawyers.[5] Equally, where an employee is injured at work the courts may hold an accepted industrial practice to be negligent.[6]

The courts have taken a different view in medical cases, where compliance with professional practice is, as a matter of law, *not* negligent.[7] Medical men are, therefore, put in a very favourable position. While the law imposes a duty of care, uniquely the medical profession sets its own standard of care. Schiemann J. only denied the application of the latter part of *Bolam*.

The exceptional rule exists because a judge is not in a position to "second guess" the expert evidence about the propriety of the treatment or diagnosis. What should perhaps have been only "a rule of thumb," reflecting the practical limitation on judicial capacity to evaluate expert evidence, has become a rule of law. Other jurisdictions have not accepted this shift of emphasis, for example, in Canada,[8] Australia[9] and, even, the occasional English judge has been tempted to be less respectful of expert evidence.[10] However, in view of *Whitehouse* and *Maynard* it does not seem that the courts, in England, are not at liberty to take such an approach in cases of negligent treatment or diagnosis.

The "Bolam Test" and Sidaway

Lloyd L.J. relied on the speech of Lord Diplock in *Sidaway* as deciding that *Bolam* applied to cases of medical advice as well as treatment and diagnosis. While all the Law Lords in *Sidaway* dismissed the plaintiff's appeal, their reasons for doing so differed. Was Lord Diplock's view, so heavily relied upon by Lloyd L.J., shared by the other Law Lords? Undoubtedly, Lord Diplock took the most conservative view of the judicial role in evaluating expert evidence when he applied *Bolam*. He alone of the Law Lords was content to leave the scope of a doctor's duty of disclosure to the medical profession itself. In a lecture delivered in 1985,[11] Lord Scarman put Lord Diplock's view of the law in perspective. He said

"We can ignore Lord Diplock's opinion, as he was in a minority of one; the other three opinions were perhaps truer to the spirit of English law."

As we have seen Lord Bridge (with whom Lord Keith agreed) and Lord Templeman, did not take the same view of the law as Lord Diplock. These judges would not consider compliance with professional practice as necessarily determinative of the question of negligence.

The "Bolam Test" and Contraceptive Advice

If, as we have seen, the courts will now consider professional practice negligent in some circumstances, could the failure to disclose risks and alternatives in the contraceptive context be one? Schiemann J. thought that it was. But, in the Court of Appeal Lloyd L.J. attacked the linchpin of Schiemann J.'s judgment—the *therapeutic/non-therapeutic* distinction. He rejected the distinction because it was vague and elusive. This is no reason for throwing out distinctions altogether, many legal notions are vague and elusive, for example, reasonable foreseeability in tort—that is often the nature of the beast.

The 'therapeutic' nature, which is at the heart of most medical procedures, is central to the *Bolam* test. The court in *Sidaway* was anxious not to trespass on the medical profession's "therapeutic privilege" to act in the best interests of the health of the patient. Lord Scarman accepted this, even though he totally abandoned the "*Bolam* test," preferring the more onerous duty of disclosure of the "reasonable or prudent patient" accepted in some North American jurisdictions.[12] The difference between the views of Lord Bridge and Lord Scarman is probably only one of burden of proof. In advice cases, Lord Scarman would place the burden on the doctor to justify his "therapeutic privilege" to withhold information in the patient's health interests. Lord Bridge, on the other hand, saw "therapeutic privilege" as an integral part of any "competent body of medical opinion" which would take this issue into account.

Neither judge's premise would, on its face, justify the doctor withholding information in a contraceptive case where the treatment is being sought for financial or social reasons. There is nothing to weigh in the balance against disclosure. As Lord Scarman recently said in an article in which he explained the effect of the *Sidaway* decision:[13]

> "if there are no medical reasons which should be operative against informing your patient as to the consequences of the operation you are proposing, the doctor is obliged by law to give an explanation of those consequences, the cons as well as the pros, to his patient."

A little later in the article the judge continues[14]

> "*Sidaway* reveals that, save in exceptional circumstances, a patient has a right to know the risks as well as the advantages of the treatment proposed and the alternative options to the treatment proposed."

It cannot be denied that medical skill is required in sterilisation cases: (a) to know the risks and alternatives to the procedure and (b) to assess the patient's condition in order to determine whether the patient's health will be affected by knowledge of the risks, to carry out the procedure itself and to determine the consequences for the patient if nothing is done. But, all this justifies is *reference* to medical practice without *deference* to it. Notwithstanding what Lloyd L.J. said, this is precisely the approach Schiemann J. took at first instance.

Of course, it might be different, if the sterilisation operation was also for therapeutic reasons as, for example, in *Jones* v. *Berkshire A.H.A.*[15] where there was a risk to the patient's health if she became pregnant again. But, even in this circumstance how can any "therapeutic discretion" excuse a doctor from informing a patient of alternatives. If the fear is that the patient will forgo any treatment if told the truth, is that fear really well-founded in this situation? It is interesting to note that in *F.* v. *R.*[16] King C.J. said

> "If there had been a medically acceptable choice between tubal ligation with a slight risk of failure and another medically acceptable operation with no risk of failure, I would have held that there was a duty to volunteer full information to enable an intelligent choice to be made."

But since, usually, contraception will be sought for economic or social reasons as in *Udale*, there is no reason to have a rule which elevates "professional skill" to pride of place, when rarely beyond the initial stages of any consultation will it be relevant.

A month after *Gold* was decided, the Court of Appeal in *Palmer* v. *Eadie*[17] reached the same conclusion applying *Sidaway* but, curiously, without reference to *Gold*. The court came to the view that a doctor had not been negligent in failing to discuss the alternative methods of vasectomy with the plaintiff. This was in accordance with the practice of the profession and, therefore, "whether on the basis of Lord Bridge's approach, Lord Diplock's approach or Lord Templeman's approach" there was no negligence.[18]

3. *Causation*

Even if the plaintiff can establish that the doctor had been negligent in failing to inform him there will often be insuperable difficulties in establishing that the failure to inform caused him any harm. The plaintiff can put forward one of two arguments. First that as a result of the failure to inform the patient of the risks of natural reversal of the sterilisation operation, he would not have consented to it; as was argued in *Gold*. Secondly, as in *Thake*, the patient might argue that although she would have undergone the procedure, had she known of the risk of failure, she would have been put on notice of the risk of becoming pregnant and so would have more readily noticed her pregnancy and so could have sought an abortion to avoid the birth.

It is central to this species of the action that the patient would have either, in the first situation, refused the procedure or, in the second situation, undergone an abortion. Without proof of this the patient will not be able to show that the doctor's negligent non-disclosure caused the injury and loss suffered. On what basis is this hypothetical decision determined? Is the question here, what would *the patient* have done if he or she had known of the risk of failure (a subjective causation requirement) or, instead, what would *the reasonable man or woman* in the patient's position have done (an objective causation requirement)?

(a) *The Objective Test Abroad*

In both Canada[19] and America[20] the courts have opted for the objective test because of the dangers of relying on the patient's views in hindsight after injury or harm has been suffered of what they would have done before the injury or harm occurred. As Linden J. put it in the Canadian case of *White* v. *Turner*[21]

> "It is not enough . . . for the court to be convinced that the plaintiff would have refused the treatment if he had been fully informed; the Court must *also* be satisfied that a reasonable patient, in the same situation would have done so."

Adopting an objective test (and applying *Canterbury*) in a case of a failed sterilisation, the Maryland's Court of Appeal in *Sard* v. *Hardy*[22] stated that if the subjective test applied

> "the testimony of the plaintiff as to what he would have hypothetically done would be the controlling consideration. Thus, proof of causation . . . would ultimately turn on the credibility of the hindsight of a person seeking recovery after he had experienced a most undesirable result . . . Under [an objective test], the patient's hindsight as to what he would have hypothetically done, though relevant, is not determinative of the issue."

In both Canada and America, the objective causation test has limited the liability of the medical profession even though these jurisdictions recognise that a greater degree of disclosure is essential for a doctor to fulfil his legal obligations.[23] There is no doubt that causation would (and does) play equally as important a role in England in limiting professional liability.

(b) *The Subjective Test in England*

In England, the relative merits of the objective and subjective tests have never been examined. What case law there is seems to adopt a subjective approach. But this should not lead you to think that patients fare any better than they do in North America. In *Chatterton* v. *Gerson*[24] the plaintiff consented to an injection to relieve the pain caused by a hernia. The doctor failed to disclose the risk that the procedure might cause the loss of sensation in her right leg. In determining whether the patient would have consented if she had known of this risk, Bristow J. looked to the patient's choice.

However, this case illustrates that the fear of the North American courts that the patient's evidence would be determinative is ill-founded. Bristow J. determined on the facts that, notwithstanding her evidence that she would have refused the operation, he was satisfied, on a balance of probabilities, that she would have undergone it even had she known of the risk.

Chatterton was, of course, a case concerned with therapeutic treatment as, indeed, have been the majority of the cases where the court has rejected the plaintiff's evidence about what they would have done. The court has regard to the fact that the plaintiff might have been in pain, was anxious to do something about a troublesome ailment and might have been in need of some treatment. Often these considerations will be absent in the case of sterilisation procedures, especially if they are done solely for social or economic reasons. We might, therefore, expect judges to be more ready to believe a plaintiff when he or she says "if I had known there was a failure rate I would not have consented to the procedure."

However, in the case where the issue is whether the patient would have refused outright any contraceptive treatment if a very small risk of reversal had been mentioned, it is likely that the courts will view the patient's evidence with the same scepticism as Bristow J. did the plaintiff's in *Chatterton*.

The position might be different if there is a viable alternative procedure with a lower failure rate. In *Gold* v. *Haringay H.A.*, the trial judge[25] found that if the possibility of a vasectomy had been mentioned to the patient, then she would not have undergone the sterilisation operation, but instead, her husband would have had the vasectomy. The judge came to this view notwithstanding the fact that subsequent to the birth of the child who was the subject of the action the husband had not had a vasectomy and, indeed, the Golds had produced another child. In some cases, a court might come to a different conclusion because of the therapeutic nature of the sterilisation operation which, as with all such procedures, may well incline a court to the view that the patient would not have refused the treatment undertaken.

A plaintiff's evidence is likely to be more cogent if the issue is whether the non-disclosure deprived the patient of the opportunity of an abortion because, this too, can be seen as a viable alternative if there are any medical or psychiatric grounds for the abortion. In *Thake* v. *Maurice*,[26] the Court of Appeal upheld the trial judge's finding that Mrs Thake could (and would) have had an abortion had she been on guard to spot the signs of pregnancy, if she had thought it was possible after a sterilisation operation.

In the end, it may not matter whether the courts adopt a subjective or an objective test of causation. Even if the test is subjective, as *Chatterton* illustrates, the judges seem to adopt a yardstick of reasonableness as an evidentiary tool with which to assess the plaintiff's evidence. Unreasonable claims lose either way.

E. *Conclusion*

The Court of Appeal in *Gold* was anxious to limit the availability of negligence actions for failed sterilisations. The Court of Appeal seems to have been uneasy in awarding damages for the birth of a healthy child which would make the doctor the "financial father" of the child. Perhaps, Lloyd L.J. did not agree with the Court of Appeal in *Emeh* v. *Kensington and Chelsea A.H.A.*,[27] that it was not contrary to public policy to award damages for maintaining the child to majority.

The recognition of a duty to disclose should not be seen merely as a means of compensating unwanted parenthood. If doctors disclosed more information a franker and fuller dialogue between doctor and patient would result. Indeed, there would be nothing for a patient to complain about if he has made an "informed" choice.

If the dislike of *Emeh* underlies the decision in *Gold*, subject to the doctrine of *stare decisis*, is this not a case of the "tail wagging the dog"? Which is the better solution: an extensive recovery of damages with a narrow area of liability or a restricted recovery of damages in a wider area of liability? Which do you think would better serve the patient's "right to know?"

Notes

[1] *Baker* v. *Bolton* (1808) 1 Camp. 493; *Osborn* v. *Gillett* (1873) L.R. 8 Ex. 88; *Admiralty Commissioners* v. *S.S. Amerika* [1917] A.C. 38.
[2] Initially in 1846. Together with subsequent amendments, the law is now contained in the Fatal Accidents Act 1976 (as amended).
[3] For a most thorough analysis of the American law, see A. Capron, "Tort Liability in Genetic Counselling," (1979) 29 Columb. L.R. 618.
[4] The classic analysis of this cause of action is Tedeschi, "On Tort Liability for 'Wrongful Life' " (1966) 1 Israel L.R. 513.
[5] The leading cases are *Gleitman* v. *Cosgrove* (1967) 386 N.E.2d 807 and *Berman* v. *Allan* (1979) 404 A.2d 8. Cf. *Park* v. *Chessin* (1977) 400 N.Y.S.2d 110, overruled (1978) 413 N.Y.S.2d 895 and *Curlender* v. *Bio-Science Laboratories* (1980) 165 Cal. Rptr. 477.
[6] *Turpin* v. *Sortini* (1982) 643 P.2d 954.
[7] *Procanik* v. *Cillo* (1984) 478 A.2d 755.
[8] *Harbeson* v. *Parke-Davis Inc.* (1983) 656 P.2d 483.
[9] [1982] 2 All E.R. 771. Discussed by Weir [1982] C.L.J. 225 and Robertson (1982) 45 M.L.R. 697.
[10] See Teff, "The Action for 'Wrongful Life' in England and the United States" (1985) 34 I.C.L.Q. 423.
[11] For a criticism of these reasons, see Teff *ibid.* and Fortin, "Is the 'Wrongful Life' Action Really Dead?" [1987] J.S.W.L. 306.
[12] *McKay supra.* per Stephenson L.J. at 779; per Ackner L.J. at 787 and per Griffiths L.J. at 789. This is formidable authority but Fortin *ibid.* 311–312 argues that the statute has not had this effect. However, her argument is unconvincing.
[13] Section 1(2)(a).
[14] Is this not a "wrongful life" action which the Law Commission thought the 1976 Act would abolish? – Report No. 60 on "Injuries to Unborn Children" Cmnd. 5709 (1974) paras. 85–89. See also the Pearson Commission (1978) Cmnd. 7054 para. 1485.
[15] (1979) 123 S.J. 406 (Watkins J.) unreported in the Court of Appeal (Transcript 78/NJ/262, July 24, 1980) but noted by Robertson (1981) 44 M.L.R. 215.
[16] See especially Stephenson L.J. at 777 and Ackner L.J. at 785.
[17] See W.V.H. Rogers, "Legal Implications of Ineffective Sterilisation" (1985) 5 Legal Studies 296. For the American law see Mark, "Liability For Failure of Birth Control Methods" (1976) 76 Colum. L.R. 1187.
[18] For the problems of what exactly constitutes the injury and so "triggers" the limitation period, see Rogers *ibid.*, 309–313.

[19] Note *Pattinson* v. *Hobbs* (Court of Appeal November 5, 1985) where a vasectomy failed but the parents did not claim any damages for physical injury and the court treated their claim as one for economic loss.

[20] *The Times*, July 15, 1961.

[21] The father of the recently retired Lord Chancellor and the newly appointed Lord Justice Butler-Sloss.

[22] (Unreported decision of Crichton J. April 29, 1977). See also *Wells* v. *Surrey A.H.A.* (unreported decision of Croom-Johnson J., July 28, 1978).

[23] *Thake* v. *Maurice* [1986] 1 All E.R. 497.

[24] *Udale* v. *Bloomsbury A.H.A.* [1983] 2 All E.R. 522; *Emeh* v. *Kensington A.H.A.* [1985] 3 All E.R. 1044; *Eyre* v. *Measday* [1986] 1 All E.R. 488; *Gold* v. *Haringay H.A.* [1987] 2 All E.R. 888.

[25] See also *Jones* v. *Berkshire A.H.A.* July 2, 1986; *Venner* v. *North East Essex H.A.*, February 19, 1987; *Worster* v. *City and Hackney A.H.A.*, June 19, 1987; *Pattinson* v. *Hobbs* (*supra*); *Morris* v. *South Manchester Private Clinic*, April 29, 1986; *Palmer* v. *Eadie*, May 18, 1987.

[26] *Supra.*

[27] See also the remarks of MacPherson J. in *Morris* v. *South Manchester Private Clinic, supra*, "I am . . . spared or prevented from giving voice to my own judgment or opinion . . . which . . . might not have been exactly the same."

[28] *Supra.*

[29] See C. Symmons, "Policy Factors in Actions For Wrongful Birth," (1987) 50 M.L.R. 269—the paper considers what I prefer to call "wrongful conception" cases.

[30] In all the cases so far the damages have been low—*e.g. Udale* (*supra*) about £9,000; *Thake* (*supra*) about £11,000. But the figures are rising—*Gold* (*supra*) £19,000 and in *Jones* (*supra*) about £33,000.

[31] We have not yet had the case of the plaintiffs who wish to send their child to private school. But on what basis could a judge refuse to award the fees?

[32] [1983] 2 All E.R. 522.

[33] *Supra* text to notes 10–11.

[34] See Purchas L.J. in *Emeh supra* at 1056 citing *Sherlock* v. *Stillwater Clinic* (1977) 260 N.W.2d 169.

[35] In *Thake* v. *Maurice supra*, the Court of Appeal held this could be set-off against the time and trouble of raising a child but not against either pre-natal pain and suffering or post-natal financial claims.

[36] *Supra* at 531.

[37] [1984] 2 All E.R. 513—not questioned in the Court of Appeal.

[38] [1984] 3 All E.R. 961.

[39] Leave to appeal was refused by the House of Lords. But this should not have been taken as agreement with the Court of Appeal see, *Wilson* v. *Colchester Justices* [1985] 2 All E.R. 97, 100 *per* Lord Roskill.

[40] *Supra* at 1051; see also Slade L.J. at 1054.

[41] *Supra* at 1056.

[42] *Ibid.*

[43] See Robertson, "Civil Liability Arising from 'Wrongful Birth' Following an Unsuccessful Sterilization Operation" (1976) 4 Am. J. Law & Med. 131.

[44] *Supra.*

[45] *Supra.*

[46] Unreported Court of Appeal decision, May 18, 1987.

[47] [1980] 5 W.W.R. 273 (British Columbia Supreme Court, Bouck J.).

[48] See the explanation of this case in *F.* v. *R.* (1983) 33 S.A.S.R. 189, 194–5 *per* King C.J. and 206 *per* Bollen J.

[49] Unreported decision of Tucker J., February 19, 1987.

Conclusion

145

[50] There is no duty, usually, to disclose the obvious, see *Sidaway* v. *Bethlem Royal Hospital* [1985] 1 All E.R. 643, 644 *per* Lord Templeman. It might be different if the doctor ought to know that the patient does not know the obvious.

[51] See also *Morris* v. *South Manchester Private Clinic supra*.

[52] *Bolam* v. *Friern H.M.C.* [1957] 1 W.L.R. 582. Approved by the House of Lords in *Whitehouse* v. *Jordan* [1981] 1 W.L.R. 246; *Maynard* v. *West Midland R.H.A.* [1984] 1 W.L.R. 634.

[53] *Per* McNair J. at 587. Approved in *Maynard*. See also Lord Scarman in *Sidaway* at 649, in relation to "treatment" and "diagnosis."

[54] The plaintiff will also have to prove that the defendant's negligence caused the harm. After *Emeh* v. *Kensington and Chelsea A.H.A.* a woman's decision not to have an abortion will rarely (*per* Slade L.J.) or never (*per* Waller and Purchas L.JJ.) break the chain of causation.

[55] (1971) 187 N.W.2d 511.

[56] Again the court would apply the *"Bolam* test" to determine this.

[57] *e.g Sard* v. *Hardy* (1977) 379 A.2d 1014 (Maryland Court of Appeals).

[58] *Supra*.

[59] *e.g. Custodio* v. *Bauer* (1967) 59 Cal. Rptr. 463 (California Court of Appeal).

[60] *Supra*.

[61] *Supra*.

[62] [1986] 1 All E.R. 488.

[63] See *infra* text to notes 65–73.

[64] [1981] 1 All E.R. 257, 265. See also *Brushett* v. *Cowan* (1988) 40 D.L.R. (4th) 488.

[65] Or, of course, for negligently performing the procedure in breach of an implied term of the contract to exercise reasonable care and skill.

[66] See Bell (1984) 4 Legal Studies 175.

[67] *Supra*.

[68] *Supra*.

[69] See *Sard* v. *Hardy supra*, (no consideration for a post-operative promise). *Cf. Custodio* v. *Bauer supra*, (an express agreement to sterilise).

[70] *Supra per* Slade L.J. at 494.

[71] See also *Gold* v. *Haringay H.A. supra per* Lloyd L.J. at 896.

[72] *Supra* at 512.

[73] *Thake supra per* Nourse L.J. at 511.

[74] [1987] 1 F.L.R. 125.

[75] Paragraph 7A of the statement of claim.

[76] Unreported, June 19, 1987.

[77] *Supra*.

[78] *Supra*. See also *Grey* v. *Webster* (1985) 14 D.L.R. (4th) 706 (New Brunswick Court of Queen's Bench)—action failed on causation.

[79] [1985] 1 All E.R. 577.

[80] For a discussion, see Powell and Jackson Professional Negligence (2nd Ed.) 1987 Chap. 6.

[81] Lords Bridge, Keith and Templeman.

[82] *Supra* at 665.

[83] *Supra* at 666.

[84] *Supra* at 663.

[85] *Ibid*. Surely this is what Sir John Donaldson M.R. meant when he said the practice must be *rightly* accepted by the medical profession? [1984] 1 All E.R. 1018, 1028 (his emphasis).

[86] See the explanation by Lloyd L.J. in *Gold* at 895.

[87] See Lloyd L.J. *ibid*.

[88] (1983) 33 S.A.S.R. 189.

[89] *Ibid* at 196.

[90] See Grubb, "A Survey of Medical Malpractice Law in England: Crisis? What Crisis?" (1985) 1 J. Contemp. Health L. and Pol'y. 75, 108–110.

[91] *Lee* v. *South West Thames R.H.A.* [1985] 2 All E.R. 385, 389–390 *per* Sir John Donaldson M.R.

[92] *per* Lord Bridge in *Sidaway* at 661. See also Lord Diplock at 659 and Lord Templeman at 664.

[93] *The Times*, February 11, 1987

[94] *The Times*, May 24, 1985 (Leonard J.).

[95] Neill L.J. may have made this distinction. If so, why talk of *Bolam* since that is solely concerned with the normative question?

[96] [1987] 2 All E.R. 888. See Grubb [1988] C.L.J. 12.

[97] [1987] 1 F.L.R. 125.

[98] *Quaere* whether this is correct? See *infra* text to notes 1–10. See also *Palmer* v. *Eadie supra per* Sir Fredrick Lawton.

[99] *Supra* at 140.

[1] See generally, *Jackson and Powell*, Professional Negligence *supra*.

[2] *Supra*.

[3] *Supra*.

[4] *Lloyds Bank Ltd.* v. *Savory* [1933] A.C. 201 (H.L.).

[5] *Midlands Bank* v. *Hett, Stubbs & Kemp* [1979] Ch. 384 (Oliver J.), *Edward Wong Finance* v. *Johnson, Stokes & Master* [1984] A.C. 296 (P.C.).

[6] *Cavanagh* v. *Ulster Weaving Co. Ltd.* [1960] A.C. 145 (H.L.); *Thompson* v. *Smiths Shiprepairers (North Shields) Ltd.* [1984] Q.B. 405 (Mustill J.).

[7] *Vancouver General Hospital* v. *McDaniel* (1935) 152 T.L.R. 56 (P.C.); *Marshall* v. *Lindsey C.C.* [1935] 1 K.B. 516 (C.A.) and *Whiteford* v. *Hunter* [1950] W.N. 533 (H.L.).

[8] *Chasney* v. *Anderson* (1959) 4 D.L.R. 223.

[9] *F.* v. *R.* (1983) 33 S.A.S.R. 189.

[10] *Clark* v. *Adams* (1950) 94 S.J. 599; and *Hucks* v. *Coles*, *The Times*, May 9, 1968.

[11] (1986) 79 J. Roy. Soc. Med. 697.

[12] *e.g.* Canterbury v. *Spence* 1972) 464 F.2d 772 and *Reibl* v. *Hughes* (1980) 114 D.L.R. (3d) 1. See Grubb, *op. cit.* at 93–111.

[13] *Medicine in Contemporary Society: King's College Studies 1986–7.* (*ed. by P. Byrne*), at 131, 136.

[14] *Ibid.* at 139.

[15] *Supra*.

[16] *Supra.* at 196.

[17] Unreported May 18, 1987.

[18] *Ibid. per* Sir Frederick Lawton.

[19] In the Supreme Court Decision of *Reibl* v. *Hughes* (1980) 114 D.L.R. (3d) 1. Discussed by Robertson, "Overcoming the Causation Hurdle in Informed Consent Cases: The Principle in *McGhee* v. *N.C.B.*" (1984) 22 U.W. Ont. L.R. 75.

[20] In the influential District of Columbia case of *Canterbury* v. *Spence* (1972) 464 F.2d 772.

[21] (1981) 120 D.L.R. (3d) 269, 286.

[22] *Supra* at 1025. See also in Canada, *Grey* v. *Webster* (1985) 14 D.L.R. (4th) 706 (sterilisation operation—plaintiff established breach of duty but lost on causation).

[23] See, Dugdale (1986) 2 P.N. 108, 109–110. But not always: see *Haughian* v. *Paine* (1987) 37 D.L.R. (4th) 624 (Saskatchewan Court of Appeal).

[24] [1981] 1 All E.R. 257.

[25] [1987] 1 F.L.R. 125 (Schiemann J.).

[26] *Supra*.

[27] *Supra*.

No Fault Liability And Medical Responsibility

SHEILA McLEAN

In their evidence to the Royal Commission on Civil Liability and Compensation for Personal Injury[1] (Pearson Commission) the medical profession's representations indicated their general hostility to modification or alteration of the basis of liability for personal injury.[2] However much the fault based action may be criticised, the medical profession believed it to be "one of the means whereby doctors could show their sense of responsibility and, therefore, justly claim professional freedom."[3] Thus, their view was that—even if a change in the basis of liability was to be considered—the fault based system should continue to be an option. Not only were they concerned that professional freedom would be curtailed by an alteration in liability, but they also feared that such a state run system would permit of intrusion into and bureaucratisation of medical practice.[4] It is fair to say that the Pearson Commission was not overly impressed by such claims,[5] but they nonetheless did not recommend changes to the basis of liability.

Increasingly, however, under headlines such as "How to Remove Financial Insult from Injury"[6] the press report a change of attitude amongst the medical profession. Now, it would appear, the arguments which so failed to impress the Pearson Commission, also fail to impress the medical profession itself. The BMA is becoming a strong supporter of a no fault system. The question to be posed, therefore, is what is it that has brought about such a dramatic change in attitude? Moreover, although it is often reported that a no fault system is now actively recommended, the efficacy of such a system for the patient is seldom explored in any depth. The tacit assumption that the system simply *is* better needs, however, to be more carefully scrutinised, in the light of what it is that we seek to achieve. Massive and fundamental legal change requires justification. In this paper, therefore, I would propose to consider what might be the rationale for change, to assess the position which obtains in the world's most comprehensive no fault system—created in 1972 in New Zealand—and to assess the efficacy of liability without fault for the patient who is damaged as a result of his or her contact with medicine.

Reasons for Change

There can be little doubt that many are dissatisfied with the current situation in respect of medical injury. Whatever the reasons, patients seem to be less likely to win their case against a doctor in court,[7] litigation in any event can be protracted and expensive, not to say uncertain,[8] and, it is claimed, excessive litigation (however that is defined) leads inevitably to changes in medical practice which ultimately benefit neither doctor nor patient.[9] The reasons for change could be put thus: the increase in challenges to the medical profession means that doctors have to pay higher premiums to their defence organisations; increase in litigation will nevitably lead to the practice of defensive medicine; only the doctor whom the defence organisation feels it can defend is exposed to the trauma of litigation; and in any event, the majority of cases where patients do sustain damage are really cases of medical accident and not cases of negligence. They cannot therefore attract compensation in any event under the current system, but considerable damage may be done to the doctor/ patient relationship by attempts to raise actions. Further, if patients do need assistance they may not need financial help, and if financial help is what they need, litigation takes so long that the help is not there when they need it.

Now, of course, most of these reasons were also true when the medical profession defended the fault based system before the Pearson Commission. In fact the crucial difference between then and now is probably that, although litigation was increasing even then, it is said to be spiralling faster now. So, the central rationale for current medical support for legal change may well be doctors' fears of being sued. This, of course, need not be presented, just as a selfish fear on the part of individual doctors, but may also represent a threat to patient care. If doctors are sued more often, and more successfully, we are told, then they will increasingly practice defensive medicine, taken to imply, for example, excessive diagnostic zeal. The result of this can be to place the patient at more risk (since some diagnostic procedures are themselves highly invasive and not without risk) and to stretch the resources of the health service by undertaking unnecessary procedures. In this scenario, no one is a winner.

Even in 1978, the Pearson Commission were unimpressed by the threat of defensive medicine becoming a reality in the U.K., for reasons which are well known and theoretically convincing.[10] In addition to these standard arguments it must also be asked whether it makes any sense to assert that if negligent practices are found to be negligent then the non-negligent doctor will inevitably change his or her non-negligent practices. If on the other hand that same doctor has been acting negligently then there is no reason to be other than delighted if he or she then changes that practice. To imply anything else might seem to be a somewhat cynical view of a professional group, and if defensive medicine *is* on the increase, then we should perhaps be questioning the professionalism of the individuals concerned rather than concerning ourselves with massive and fundamental legal change. Current claims that there has been, and continues to be, a growth in defensive practice by doctors, however unnecessary, must nonetheless be taken into account at the level of practice rather than theory since the effect on medical practice and patient care is not to be underestimated.

Litigation can damage the doctor/patient relationship and it may be that some support for a relatively non-combative and uncontentious system could come from this fact alone. However, it is also clearly the case that *negligence* damages the doctor/patient relationship, as does the failure of doctors to explain honestly to patients that they have been the victims of a medical accident or of negligent or careless therapy, and yet this situation is the norm rather than the exception.

Whatever the plausibility of the threat of defensive medicine, however, there may be more convincing reasons to consider the pattern of medical litigation and the outcome of patients' grievances as unsatisfactory and in need of change. In fact, if Pearson is right, the main reason for supporting a shift in the basis for the assessment of professional liability may well be that medical accident is more common than medical negligence[11] and that therefore only by modifying legal process will the patient be compensated in the majority of cases. Change may mean that the medical profession can breathe more easily, and practice their profession without undue fear of litigation, and the patient will be in a position to obtain much needed assistance in dealing with the potentially far-reaching consequences of harm suffered.

At first sight, a system of liability which does not depend on proof of fault seems to offer the solution to many of the dissatisfactions with the current system of liability. Certainly it seems to be the case that its value is relatively uncritically assumed by the media, and perhaps even by the public and the medical profession also. It may seem somewhat paradoxical in these days of free enterprise and retrenchment in state intervention that the lobby in favour of what is a state funded compensation scheme is gaining support—but perhaps this merely reflects the power and credibility of the profession who have now thrown their weight behind it. And, of course, if it is the case that a no fault system provides ready access to compensation and avoids the threat of defensive medicine, then the fact that it may seem somewhat out of line with current political thinking may be interesting, but can scarcely be of ultimate importance.

The next part of this paper, will look at the operation of the no fault system in New Zealand and consider its effects on medical responsibility and the rights of patients. The aim is to assess the extent to which this particular system can in theory achieve what is sought, and to consider whether or not it does so in practice. If the reasons for change are to remove the threat of litigation from doctors, whilst at the same time enhancing patient care and respecting patients' rights and needs, and to provide relevant, speedy and appropriate compensation for those damaged by medical care, then the question to be answered is the extent to which the system can or does provide this.

No Fault in New Zealand

Inevitably, in any scheme, whether or not it equates to a kind of social security system, the first concern is to define eligibility. Eligibility has, unfortunately, proved to be one of the major problems of the New Zealand scheme. The Accident Compensation Act 1972 set up the basic structure for the system and outlined the basis for eligibility, and the amendments subsequently made to the legislation are incorporated into consolidating legislation in the Accident Compensation Act 1982. Based on the Report of the Committee of Inquiry (Woodhouse Report)[12] the legislation also incorporated what could be described as some of the fundamental illogicalities of that report. Eligibility is based on damage resulting from "personal injury by accident" which is defined as follows:

"Personal injury by accident"—

(a) Includes—

> (i) The physical and mental consequences of any such injury or of the accident.
> (ii) Medical, surgical, dental, or first aid misadventure.
> (iii) Incapacity resulting from occupational disease or indust- rial deafness to the extent that cover extends in respect of the disease or industrial deafness . . .
> (iv) Actual bodily harm (including pregnancy and mental or nervous shock) arising by any act or omission of any other person which is within the description of any of the offences specified in sections 128, 132, and 201 of the Crimes Act 1961, irrespective of whether or not any person is charged with the offence and notwithstanding that the offender was legally incapable of forming a criminal intent.

(b) Except as provided in the last preceding paragraph, does not include—

> (i) Damage to the body or mind caused by a cardio-vascular or cerebro-vascular episode unless the episode is the result of effort, strain, or stress that is abnormal, excessive, or unusual for the person suffering it, and the effort, strain, or stress arises out of and in the course of the employment of that person.
> (ii) Damage to the body or mind caused exclusively by disease, infection, or the ageing process."[13]

Although the exclusion of sickness from eligibility reflects the views of the Woodhouse Commission, it has served to provide some of the major obstacles to the achievement of a truly equitable and wide-ranging system of liability. Indeed, it is also one of the under- lying philosophical problems of the system, which simultaneous with making such exclusions was nonetheless pledged to ensure that "all injured persons should receive compensation from any community financed scheme on the same uniform method of assessment, *regard- less of the causes which give rise to their injuries*."[14]

The vision of Woodhouse is considerably restricted by the making of such an exclusion, and it is worth noting that Mr. Justice Woodhouse, when chairing a subsequent Commission in Australia, made no such distinction between accident and disease.

At first sight, however, and even accepting that this distinction represents a flaw in the system, the definition given of personal injury by accident seems to provide a relatively straightforward basis on which to assess eligibility. The apparent simplicity, however, belies the problems which have arisen. Cripps, for example, has claimed that:

> "The meaning of "accident" for the purposes of the Act has been a fundamental problem which has not been simplified by legislative definition. However, it is clear that merely because an injury is unexpected and caused by negligence it will not necessarily be covered by the Act."[15]

In any system of liability, interpretation of key words will play a major part in deciding who should benefit. This, of course, has long been one of the problems identified with the fault based system, but it seems clear that the operation of the no fault system will not inevitably be free from similar problems. Indeed, Palmer has said that:

> "To begin with the idea was to spell everything out so people would know their rights. The trend of the amendments has been to give more and more discretion to the Commission so that certainty is lost but the obscurity remains. At present neither clarity nor predictability exist."[16]

The interpretation of "accident" was initially based on the definition given in the case of *Jones* v. *Secretary of State for Social Services*[17] and incorporated events which were unlooked for and undesigned. The Accident Compensation Corporation advised doctors that "[a]s a matter of general principle *personal injury by accident* means any form of damage to the human system which is unexpected and was not designed by the person injured."[18] However, although seemingly straightforward, interpretational variations have resulted in a lack of consistency and objectivity. Two cases show that "accident" may not be an uncomplicated concept. In the first case, it was said that "[a]ccident should be interpreted in its ordinary and popular meaning, as normally denoting an unlooked-for mishap or untoward event which is neither expected nor designed," and which is "capable of being described as occurring at some particular time rather than by gradual process."[19] Yet in another case which arose at about the same time, nothing is quite so simple. Here it was said that:

"If a happening is accidental merely because it is a happening by chance then I suppose it must be conceded that the happening is an accident but only to the extent that it is a chance. The daily life of every one of us is packed with chance happenings, fortuitous occurrences, coincidences, etc. of every conceivable kind. All these may be claimed by the pedants or grammarians as 'accidents' in that they occur otherwise than by design. Each is in fact a chance happening and I cannot conceive that in selecting 'accident' as the basic criterion for the operation of the Accident Compensation Act the legislature intended that the word embrace all chance happenings. I would regard the argument that as virtually all accidents are chance happenings therefore all the chance happenings of everyday life are accidents as fallacious."[20]

It does not seem unduly harsh to describe this reasoning as somewhat tortuous, but it shows an even more fundamental problem, and that is the desire—purportedly with the backing of legislative intention—to exclude some cases from the system. Interestingly, the exclusion would seem to be sought partly on the basis of the cause of the damage, yet the system was committed to compensating on the basis of the *consequences* of an accident, not its cause. Problems in reaching agreement on what is an "accident" therefore beset the system. However, for some individuals, this problem is compounded by the difficulty of distinguishing between accident and sickness. In some cases, this can be highly problematic and may result in the making of decisions which seem somewhat arbitrary, and perhaps even to be dependent on the desire to exclude on grounds which are theoretically irrelevant to the scheme—for example on policy or economic grounds. Yet such choices have to be made—however problematic they may be. As was said in one appeal case:

"The boundary line between an accident injury and a disease injury may be hard to discern at times but there is no doubt that the legislature requires the line to be drawn and the interpreter of the Act must take cognisance of this."[21]

Nowhere is the distinction between accident and illness more problematic than in cases where the claimant was already ill before the "accident." It is clear that, where such a difficulty arises, the balance is tipped in favour of illness rather than accident, and compensation is therefore precluded.[22] The exclusion of sickness is evidently one major problem faced by the New Zealand patient, but this of course need not be the case. It is a function of the particular approach adopted, and scarcely presents an insurmountable criticism of the concept of liability without fault.

A second major criticism of the New Zealand system relates to the attitude of decision-makers. Eligibility in medical cases requires evidence of 'misadventure'—this is said to be wider than negligence and to avoid many of the value judgments inherent in the terminology of fault. It has already been seen that the need to distinguish between harm caused by sickness and harm caused by accident poses particular problems in medical cases. However, if we leave this to the side for a moment, it may be the case that a wide definition of medical misadventure would serve to expand the groups for whom compensation can be sought successfully. Medical misadventure was defined as arising when "(a) a person suffers bodily or mental injury or damage in the course of, and as part of, the administering to that person of medical aid, care or attention, and (b) such injury or damage is caused by mischance or accident, unexpected and undesigned, in the nature of a medical error or medical mishap."[23] Nowhere in this definition is negligence mentioned, and indeed it is clear in that the definition is intended to cover a wider range than would negligence. Thus, medical accident could in theory be covered. This will, however, depend on the interpretation given to medical error or medical mishap.

Medical Error

This was defined in one leading review decision substantially in these terms—medical error amounts to a failure to observe "a standard of care and skill reasonably to be expected of"[24] the doctor. As the tribunal said "The test may be considered similar to the test of negligence in the common law system, but it is not intended that they should necessarily coincide."[25] However, as one commentator points out,[26] although it may not be intended that the two should coincide, the Accident Compensation decision-makers have placed a restrictive interpretation on the phrase "medical misadventure" thereby denying a number of deserving claimants compensation under the scheme.

Mahoney, in fact, is under no misapprehension that the system as currently operated serves to limit eligibility in a radical way. As he says:

"The effect...of the present interpretation of the 'medical misadventure' style of 'personal injury by accident' is blatantly ironic. Except in the unusual case of equipment failure or a bizarre and novel reaction to treatment, the person who suffers a personal injury from medical treatment must prove *fault* in the nature of 'old style' medical negligence if he hopes to receive compensation. If he cannot meet this requirement then he is denied assistance from a system that purports to have as its philosophical underpinning the abolition of the elusive search for fault."[27]

Indeed it is clear from decisions such as *Re Munday*[28] and *Re Stopford*[29] that the only risks which will, if they occur, generate compensation are very remote risks.

Although Mahoney sees some very marginal signs of change in attitude,[30] it is by no means clear that interpretation will change considerably. Thus, the patient who seeks to establish that the harm complained of was the result of medical error may well be confronted with difficulties surprisingly similar to those which confront his or her counterparts in other jurisdictions.

Medical mishap

This has been defined as being a circumstance where "there is an intervention or intrusion into the administration of medical aid, care or attention of some unexpected and undesigned incident, event or circumstance of a medical nature which has harmful consequences for the patient."[31] Effectively, therefore, medical misadventure (a combination of mishap and error) can be described very much in the same terms as medical negligence. Cases of medical mishap equate fairly closely to situations, such as leaving swabs behind after surgery, or the occurrence of an unexpected risk, which might—even in those systems which maintain the concept of fault—be dealt with by the application of *res ipsa loquitur*.[32] Examples of medical error, seem very likely to be close to those which would equate to medical negligence, but with one additional problem. It is possible, albeit relatively rare, in terms of the common law for a doctor to be held to have been negligent in failing to make an accurate diagnosis, or in failing to attend a patient. In terms of the no fault scheme, and substantially because of the exclusion of illness from compensation, neither of these events would be compensable, since the harm caused to the patient can be traced to the continuation of the pre-existing illness and not the result of an event in the nature of an accident. The suggestion that either of these events should be taken as breaking the chain and constituting a new event in the nature of an accident has been dismissed by decision-makers.[33] In other words, the patient in New Zealand may find him or her self paradoxically less likely to obtain compensation than his or her counterpart in less radical legal systems.

The patient, therefore, is left in these circumstances with only the option of raising an action through the civil courts, and on the traditional basis of negligence. Whilst it has been suggested that dissatisfaction with the level of awards made by the Accident Compensation Corporation may cause people to use this residual right of action, they may equally be deterred from so doing by the philosophy of the system itself and by the fact that their claim has already been rejected by one tribunal. As Mahoney says:

> "The very existence of the Accident Compensation Act must have a negative effect on the public's recognition of the possibility of these claims. A public that has been told for a decade that the drunk driver and the rapist are immune from civil suit can hardly be expected to learn by osmosis from a few legal journals the possibility of suing a doctor where medical treatment does not turn out as expected or promised."[34]

Consent and No Fault

It is of course true to say that the problems outlined above are not inevitably the concomitant of a no fault system, but are merely concomitant of this particular scheme. Certainly illness need not be excluded, and it is clear that decision-makers could adopt a radical rather than a restrictive interpretation of medical misadventure. Indeed, in the latter case, it may be that the intrusion of what Palmer calls "a ring of the old tort law"[35] into decision-making in medical cases may simply have reflected an old-fashioned reluctance, a hangover from the common law, to find doctors to have caused harm to their patients. Indeed, it is clearly not in the interests of the medical profession themselves that such a restrictive interpretation should be maintained, since this leaves them vulnerable to civil suit. The possibility of raising an action through the courts remains once the Accident Compensation Corporation has decided that the harm complained of does not amount to personal injury by accident, and New Zealand doctors are still recommended to maintain membership of a defence organisation.

One problem, however, which *is* central to the nature of the scheme itself, is how, if at all, the no fault approach could deal with failure to demonstrate respect for the patient's right to self-determination sufficiently by compensating in the event of inadequate disclosure of risks and benefits and alternatives in therapy.

Partly, the issue of information disclosure—as with the interpretation of medical accident or misadventure—can be affected by decision-making practices. Indeed, there is little doubt that in New Zealand it is so affected. The proposals of the Woodhouse Commission were designed to ensure that compensation was appropriate after an event which caused harm and which was unexpected or unlooked for by the person to whom the harm occurred.[26] Therefore, the patient who is not informed of possible risks would be able to claim that, if a risk actually transpires, the event was unexpected and was therefore compensable under the scheme. However, as one review case put it:

"In relation to many forms of medical or surgical treatment there are known complications or consequences and some of them may, when they occur, be unexpected by the patient although anticipated by the doctor or surgeon."[37]

That the patient did not know of the possible risks is not, however, taken to mean that the risk was unexpected and therefore compensable. Decision-makers have chosen to hold that, since the risk was known to the doctor, it was not unexpected and therefore it does not amount to personal injury by accident. Therefore, the patient will not be compensated under the accident compensation scheme unless the risk which eventuated was so rare or remote as to be unanticipated even by the doctor. There is no incentive therefore for the development of anything approaching a meaningful doctrine of consent based on information disclosure. Now, of course, this interpretation could be changed, but one further problem remains, and this one *is* central to the nature of the scheme.

The patient who claims to have been inadequately informed of risks, or alternatives, may under the common law have a claim essentially based on the insult to integrity caused by such a failure.[38] Admittedly damages might be minimal, and admittedly such claims seem to succeed relatively rarely. However, under the Accident Compensation Scheme no compensation whatsoever would be feasible. Compensation is paid substantially on the basis of lost earnings, since both the design of the scheme and the role of the state as paymaster were largely justified by the state's need to maintain a healthy work-force. There is no compensation available for insult to integrity unless it results in an inability to work for the required period. Whilst other jurisdictions struggle their way towards protection of patient autonomy in medicine (however ineffectually) the New Zealand system by its very nature can make no such moves. Whilst much of the criticism of the concept of a no fault system can be dismissed as merely reflecting an old-fashioned distaste for a scheme which does not hand out huge sums of money, but rather bases compensation on needs, or as relating to characteristics which are peculiar to *this* scheme and not the concept of no fault itself, this particular criticism is less easily defeated.

The crucial distinction between strict liability and no fault is the identity of the person or organisation funding compensation awards. Perhaps as a result of medical fears, the current vanguard of support for legal change is not support for a system of strict liability, although this would, of course, ensure that medical accidents as well as medical negligence could be compensated. The desire is, rather, to remove the burden of payment from the medical profession and on to the state—that is the cries for change (however much they purport to be in the interests of patients) are demands that the state should pay when medicine goes wrong. Inevitably, the state will place restrictions on the type of harm which can attract compensation, and even if states avoid some of the pitfalls of the system as operated in New Zealand, it seems unlikely that a demand for compensation for insult to integrity would find much support. The inability of the scheme to reinforce what is seen by many as an essential aspect of a moral medical act, and to offer some form of sanction where this is breached, is not an insignificant criticism.

Conclusion

In sum, therefore, the introduction of a no fault system may not be the unmixed blessing which it is often assumed to be. It is certainly the case that, on the positive side, claims are dealt with more speedily and that they do not involve the claimant in vast financial outlay. Moreover, the Accident Compensation Corporation estimates that the vast majority of claims *are* settled.[39] However, the residual temptation to protect the medical profession, which is said by some to be a feature of the fault based system, does seem to have a part to play in the no fault scheme also. Not only does this deny patients access to speedy, periodically reassessed and relevant compensation but it also leaves the doctor at common law risk, although certainly patients may be deterred from pursuing a claim through the courts when they have already tried and failed in one system.[40]

Nonetheless, such problems could be overcome by not adopting the classification of eligibility used in New Zealand, and by radical and liberal decision-making. However, questions relating to information disclosure, and injuries as a result of medical intervention which are not so serious as to merit reasonably lengthy absences from work, raise problems which are apparently intimately linked to the nature of the system itself rather than to anything which is susceptible of attitudinal or structural change.

It should, however, be said that our conclusions as to the value and efficacy of a no fault approach will ultimately depend on what it is that we believe a system of compensation should seek to achieve. And our conclusions on this may well hinge on our capacity to reassess the concept of compensation and traditional presuppositions about its aims. The disadvantages for certain patients, for example in matters of failure to treat or diagnose correctly, or inadequate disclosure of information, may be thought to be outweighed by the potential for speedy, needs related social assistance. Adherence to traditional thinking and concentration on the importance of certain aspects of the doctor/patient relationship may well block the path towards a more equitable scheme and a more worthwhile and appropriate distribution of resources. For this reason, such attitudes should be carefully scrutinised and analysed. Equally, however, the rationale for change must be closely scrutinised, and the extent to which patients (rather than doctors) will truly benefit from it must not be taken as read. Before fundamental legal change is seriously contemplated, and given the manifest shortcomings of liability without fault, might we not consider alternative ways of improving the current system?

Just as attitudinal and structural changes could improve the no fault scheme, so too the fault based system could benefit from such analysis. Indeed, it is a surprising but plausible conclusion that the fault based approach could perhaps encapsulate all of the legitimate grievances of patients, whilst the no fault scheme probably could not. If the movement for change is genuinely committed to improving the position of the aggrieved patient, then changes in process rather than decision making may not be the only or even the best way to achieve this.

Notes

1 Cmnd 7054/1978.
2 Pearson Report, *supra cit.*, para. 1342.
3 *Id.*
4 *Id.*
5 Para. 1343: "We record these views as put to us, although some of us feel that they are unsound and at the least overstated."
6 *The Independent*, March 17, 1987.
7 The Pearson Report, *supra cit.*, para 1326: "The proportion of successful claims for damages in tort is much lower for medical negligence than for all negligence cases. Some payment is made in 30–40 per cent. of claims compared with 86 per cent. of all personal injury claims."
8 For discussion, see e.g. Ison, T., *The Forensic Lottery*, (1967), Staples Press.
9 The claim here is that spiralling litigation will inevitably result in the practice of "defensive medicine." The Pearson Report, *supra cit.*, records in para. 1322 that "In evidence to us DHSS referred to defensive medicine, pointing to 'the rapid growth of requests for diagnostic work in both pathology and radiology, not all of which is equally productive . . . a great deal . . . is directed towards eliminating the risk of litigation in case a diagnosis is missed.' " For an alternative view of defensive medicine, see some of the contributions in C. Wood, (ed.), *The Influence of Litigation on Medical Practice*, (1977), Academic Press.
10 For a brief exposition, see the Pearson Report, *supra cit.*, para. 1323.
11 para. 1331.
12 *Compensation for Personal Injury in New Zealand*, report of the Royal Commission of Inquiry, December 1967.
13 Accident Compensation Act 1982, s.2.
14 Woodhouse Report, *supra cit.*, p. 39, para. 55.
15 C.R. Cripps, "Medical Practitioners' Liability for Personal Injury Caused by Negligence" [1978] N.Z.L.J. 83, at 84.
16 G.W.R. Palmer, "Accident Compensation in New Zealand: The First Two Years" (1977) 25 *American Journal of Comparative Law* 1 at 9.
17 [1972] All E.R. 145.
18 *Medical Information Bulletin* No. 13, October 1981.
19 Review No. 74/RO298.
20 Review No. 75/RO461.
21 Appeal Dec. No. 9 (1976).
22 *Cf.* Blair, A.P., *Accident Compensation in New Zealand*, (1978), Butterworths at 33: "If the medical evidence is in such terms as to leave the Commission with the impression that, as between accident and disease, the scales are evenly balanced, then it cannot be successfully contended that the condition laid down by the statute has been met, and the claim for compensation is therefore not established."
23 Review No. 77/R1352.
24 *Id.*

25 *Id.*

26 Mahoney, R., "Informed Consent and Breach of the Medical Contract to Achieve a Particular Result: Opportunities for New Zealand's Latent Personal Injury Litigators to Peek Out of the Accident Compensation Closet" (1985) *6 Otago Law Review*, No. 1, 103.

27 *loc.cit.*, at 107.

28 [1984] 4 N.Z.A.R. 339.

29 [1984] N.Z.A.C.R. 783.

30 Following the judgment in *MacDonald* v. *The Accident Compensation Corporation*, (unreported), High Court, Administrative Division, Hamilton, July 25, 1985, 55/85, discussed in Mahoney, *loc.cit.*

31 Review No. 77/R1352.

32 The facts speak for themselves.

33 *Cf.* Review No. 76/R1788: "The argument that interference with the natural course of things is enough to constitute internal events of this kind "accidents" is not, in my view, sound. Where such interference is carried out by persons of professional status and at the request of the patient, and where the outcome is a reasonably contemplated risk of treatment the concept of accident is quite out of place."

34 Mahoney, *loc.cit.*, at 137.

35 Palmer, *loc.cit.*, at 39.

36 *c.f.* Medical Information Bulletin, *supra cit.*

37 Review No. 75/RO236.

38 For a full discussion of the options available see M.M. Shultz, "From Informed Consent to Patient Choice: A New Protected Interest" (1985) 95 Yale Law J. 219.

39 *per* Sandford, K.L., "Personal Injury By Accident" [1980] N.Z.L.J. 29, at 30: "The percentage of claims declined is less than four per cent. and in a proportion of those the reason for declinature in some matter irrelevant to the present subject (*e.g.* that the accident happened before April 1, 1974)."

40 For discussion, see Mahoney, *loc.cit.*; see also Klar, L.N., "New Zealand's Accident Compensation Scheme: A Tort Lawyer's Perspective," (1983) 33 Univ. of Toronto Law J., 80.

INDEX

163

Index

Index

Nature,
    and science, 26
Nazis,
    and sterilisation, 5, 58–59
Necessity, doctrine of, 86
Negligence, 121–146
    Bolam test, 136–139
    and no-fault liability, 147–161
Netherlands,
    and euthanasia, 3, 112
Neville, R., 74, 76
New Zealand,
    no-fault compensation, 3, 148, 150–161
No-fault liability, 147–161
    in New Zealand, 150–161
Nozick, R., 71, 73, 77

Oakley, A., 42
O'Brien, M., 38
Ovum donation, 4, 28, 32
    between sisters, 2
Owen, Dr David, 59

Palmer, G., 152–156
Parthenogenesis, 29
Paternalism, 4, 61–62, 73–74, 110
Patient,
    age of, 106, 116–117
    to be viewed as a whole, 104–105
    some examples, 105
Pearson report, 147, 148, 149, 160
Perpetuities, law of, 2
Person, 5
    loss of and compensation, 121
POST, 31
Powell, E., 34
Precedent, role of law of, 2
Privacy, 24
Public policy, 124–126

Quinlan, Karen, 3

Rawls, J., 70, 74, 76, 77
Reid, Lord, 2, 6
Reproduction,
    political economy of, 39–41
    and discrimination, 43–45
Reproductive technologies, 23–54
    and "brave new world", 27–29
    and conflict, 25–26
    and oppression of women, 26–27, 37–38
Rights, 5

Rights—*cont.*
    absolute, 77
    and dignity, 74–75
    and reproduction, 5, 45–46, 70–77
    importance of, 71–72
    inalienable, 69–70
    justification of, 71–74
    of embryo, 10, 12–15
    of father, 55
    of mentally handicapped, 70–77
    patient's to know truth, 109–111
    to inherit, 10
    trumping of, 77
Roberts, D., 34
Roos, P., 80
Rose, N., 24, 27, 40
Rowland, R., 18, 47
Royal prerogative, 85–102
    origins, 89–93
    ideal or dormant? 95–97
Rutter, M., 44
Rust, J., 44–45

Savage, W., 38
Scarman, Lord, 138
Schiterman, B., 40
Sex selection, 28, 47
Sexuality,
    policing of, 23–25, 43–46
    and sterilisation, 55–84
Shockley, W., 83
Sign Manual, 92, 97, 101
Slippery slope argument, 19, 77–78
Social Darwinism, 57
Sotos syndrome case, 59–60, 61, 62, 63–64, 70, 71
Spencer, A., 44
Spencer, H., 79
Stanworth, M., 29
Statutory Licensing Authority, 15, 35, 36, 37
Steptoe, P., 18, 30
Sterilisation,
    failed, 2, 124–143
    of mentally handicapped, 55–84
    historical context, 56–60
    therapeutic and non-therapeutic, 62–64, 67
    and leave of court, 64
    of adult, 64–66
    and "best interests", 67–70
Suicide, 103
Surrogacy, 1, 2, 3, 28, 55
    Baby M., 3